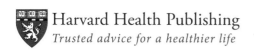
Harvard Health Publishing
Trusted advice for a healthier life

MW01195754

Dear Reader,

When you face big decisions in life, it always helps to think ahead. Can you afford to buy a new car or a home? When can you afford to retire? Where will you live after you retire? Yet many people shy away from one very important question: what type of medical care do they want if they have a chronic illness, or if they're too sick, confused, or injured to voice their wishes? Surprisingly, only 37% of Americans have documented their desires for care in the event of serious illness. Even among people ages 65 and older, only 46% have completed advance directives—documents that enable you to outline your wishes while you are still able to do so.

When the sun is shining and life is busy, it's all too easy to sidestep thoughts of debilitating injury or death. But while you may be in robust health today, you might suffer an emergency tomorrow, such as a car accident or a stroke, or you might be temporarily disabled. Or you might be diagnosed with a severe, life-threatening illness. At the very least, most of us will eventually experience declining health—which, at the end, could leave us unable to make important decisions.

At that point, if you haven't engaged in advance care planning, medical choices will be left to worried relatives, a doctor, or a guardian appointed by a judge, none of whom may have a clear understanding of your values, beliefs, and preferences. Do they know what makes life worthwhile to you—physically, emotionally, spiritually, and intellectually? What would matter most to you during your final weeks or months or if you were in the throes of a progressive, ultimately fatal illness? What kind of care would you want to receive?

The information in this Special Health Report can help you ponder and answer many of these questions before a crisis occurs. After you read it, think about your preferences. Then talk to your primary care doctor and your loved ones about what's possible and what feels right for you. These can be difficult conversations to have, but most people find it a relief to know they have voiced their wishes and laid the groundwork for decision making. It's also vital to consider who might represent your wishes (and not their own, no matter how well-meaning) should you be unable to speak for yourself.

Many of us will develop a serious illness at some point, and all of us will die one day. That's a basic truth. Ultimately, this report is about how you choose to live—all the way to the end.

Sincerely,

Muriel R. Gillick, MD

Muriel Gillick, M.D.
Medical Editor

Charles Sabatino

Charles Sabatino, J.D.
Legal Editor

Harvard Health Publishing | Harvard Medical School | 4 Blackfan Circle, 4th Floor | Boston, MA 02115

What is advance care planning?

It's not something that anyone wants to deal with, but imagine that you or a loved one has a serious progressive illness, such as multiple sclerosis or Parkinson's disease. As you age, you become less and less able to communicate your wishes. Who will speak for you? And will that person direct your health care providers to offer you the kind of care you would have asked for on your own? That is the focus of advance care planning.

Advance care planning is the process of preparing for possible future illness and incapacity by thinking in advance about what matters to you. These concerns can powerfully shape what medical treatments are right for you and, hence, what treatments you ultimately receive. Sometimes advance care planning relates to a future health state that is rare but devastating if it occurs, such as a serious accident causing head injury and coma, a persistent vegetative state, or profound cognitive dysfunction. Sometimes it addresses a future health state that is common with aging and in which many people would want medical care to be limited in some ways, such as dementia. And sometimes it focuses on a common complication or worsening of a chronic condition with which you have already been diagnosed and that you would want to be handled in a particular way.

There are multiple steps to advance care planning:
- clarifying your current health status
- thinking about and prioritizing your goals for care
- designating a surrogate decision maker (a health care agent or proxy)
- conveying your wishes to the nurses, doctors, and other health care providers caring for you, as well as to your health care proxy, often by using a form or another means (such as an audio or video recording, an online registry, a letter, a medical order signed by you and your physician, or simply a note in your medical record documenting the substance of a conversation).

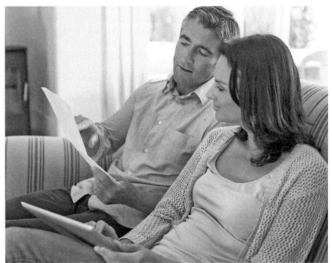

© shapecharge | Getty Images

It's tempting to think that only the very elderly or infirm need advance directives, but that's not the case. An accident could change your health status overnight.

Medicare now reimburses physicians and other qualified health professionals for discussing advance care planning with their patients. The discussion can occur at your annual wellness visit or any regular medical visit. These conversations are well worth having. Nearly a third of the Medicare budget now goes for care in the last year of life. Yet the medical care provided doesn't always lead to recovery or even comfort people in their final days. And despite the huge, positive implications for quality of life during a debilitating illness or at the end of life, many Americans fail to take advantage of advance care planning. This Special Health Report will help ensure that you are not one of them.

What are advance directives?

Advance directives are instruments that translate your wishes into documents. They allow you to describe what kind of medical care you hope to receive if an accident or illness renders you unable to communicate. In this chapter, we discuss two well-known advance directives—the health care power of attorney and the living will. We also explain two medical orders used to implement the wishes of patients with life-limiting, progressive illness or frailness—the do-not-resuscitate order (DNR) and a newer approach called POLST (physician orders for life-sustaining treatment), which a growing number of states endorse for people with certain life-limiting conditions.

Some people worry that filling out these documents means giving up control over their medical treatment. In reality, advance directives help you *gain* a measure of control over your health care. Advance directives enable you to choose the person who will make medical decisions for you when you are unable to do so—and someone will surely do this, whether or not you make a choice. Using directives, you may offer as much or as little guidance as you like.

Taking these steps can make a real difference. When researchers reviewed 113 studies on advance care planning, they found that this type of planning improves the quality of people's dying days. It leads to greater use of comfort care and hospice and results in fewer unwanted hospitalizations. Having advance directives is a good start, but the review, published in the journal *Palliative Medicine*, found that it was even more effective to make the documents part of a broader strategy that also includes frank conversations with caregivers or trained care planning facilitators. Together, these can go a long way toward increasing the chances that your wishes are acknowledged and followed, whether you are facing a serious, progressive illness or the end of your life.

Keep in mind:

- As long as you are able to make and communicate decisions, your word overrides anything you've written or told others. Only when you're unconscious or no longer have the capacity to make your wishes known does any advance directive swing fully into effect.

- You don't necessarily need any document beyond a health care power of attorney, which establishes your choice of an agent to speak for you when you cannot do so yourself. Your agent is required to respect your goals and priorities for treatment, in whatever manner you have made them known.

- If your medical condition improves enough for you to make and express your decisions, what you say at that time will again take precedence.

Many people wonder whether they need a lawyer to write an advance directive. While these forms are important legal documents that vary by state (see "State-specific considerations," page 25), they are not complicated. Thus, most people do not need a lawyer to fill out a health care power of attorney or a living will, although lawyers routinely write these documents as part of estate planning. But if you have unusual wishes for medical care or a particularly contentious family, you may benefit from legal advice.

What is a health care power of attorney?

A health care power of attorney is a legal document that permits you (the principal) to name a health care

---

Same concepts, different names

Just as laws vary from one state to another, the names of certain legal concepts are often different, too. Here are some of the alternate names you may hear for advance care planning documents, depending on the state where you live.

TERMS USED IN THIS REPORT	ALTERNATE NAMES
Health care power of attorney	• health care proxy form • medical power of attorney • durable power of attorney for health care • appointment of a health care representative form
Health care agent	• health care proxy (or just proxy) • surrogate • health care representative
Living will	• directive to physicians • health care declaration • medical directive
Do-not-resuscitate order (DNR)	• do-not-attempt-resuscitation order (DNAR) • allow-natural-death order (AND)
Physician orders for life-sustaining treatment (POLST)	• physician orders for scope of treatment (POST) • medical orders for life-sustaining treatment (MOLST) • medical orders for scope of treatment (MOST)

agent (sometimes called a health care proxy) who has legal authority to make medical decisions on your behalf if you are unable to make them yourself.

All adults should designate a health care agent. If you haven't chosen anyone, a relative or court-appointed guardian may be asked to make medical decisions for you. That person might not know your wishes or might not be comfortable following them. And if more than one close relative is at your bedside, the doctor may want all of them to come to a consensus before following any of their instructions. Sometimes conflicts ensue, and decisions may be delayed. For example, let's say your three adult children are there with you. Your doctor will probably want them all to agree on how to proceed before taking orders from them. But getting everyone to agree might be hard in such a stressful situation. It's best if you've already appointed one person to handle medical decisions using your wishes as a guide.

Generally, both law and medical ethics dictate that your health care agent must make decisions that he or she thinks you would have made. This means that your agent must be very familiar with your values, goals, and priorities regarding your medical treatment. That requires honest conversations (see "Talking to your health care agent," page 19), a written explanation of your wishes, or both.

Advance directives and dementia

Advance directives are legally valid only if the person completing them is a competent adult of sound mind. This means that someone in the advanced stages of Alzheimer's or another disease that causes confusion or dementia cannot legally fill out or sign these documents. This is another important reason to complete advance directives as early as possible.

If someone you love is in the early stages of such a disease, try to get him or her to fill out the forms and sign them in front of the appropriate witnesses during a time when he or she is still mentally able to understand the nature and effect of the document. By itself the diagnosis of Alzheimer's disease doesn't mean that the person lacks sufficient mental capacity to sign an advance directive. An individual who is unable to make medical decisions may still have sufficient mental capacity to appoint a health care agent.

Not completely certain about what you want? That's okay. Reading the information in this report will help. The next chapter explains treatment options and key concepts (see "Step 1: Deciding on your wishes for care," page 8). We've also created an informal document called the health decisions worksheet that can help you make choices and communicate your decisions (see page 35). Additional resources that you can find elsewhere include online tools and even a card game designed to take you through the decision-making process (see "Online tools," page 9, and "Resources," page 46). Note that your worksheet or online record is not legally binding, but it may provide more meaningful and flexible guidance than a formal, standardized living will.

What is a living will?

A living will is a document that enables you to describe your goals for medical treatment, your religious or spiritual beliefs, and your preferences regarding your medical treatment in various scenarios that may arise. This written record guides your doctors and loved ones in caring for you, should you ever be unable to communicate those wishes directly. Often, it's used to determine how aggressive you would like your medical treatments to be as the end of life nears.

Even though a living will is technically legally binding, note that all states permit health care providers to refuse to comply with a living will based on conscience or for ethical or professional reasons. They have an obligation to assist in transferring you to another provider who will comply, but that is not always possible or pleasant. Research has shown that the key determinant for having your wishes known and honored is not the existence of the document, but rather the quality of the communication process between you and your doctor and all others who may be involved in making health decisions for you. Discussing your wishes is the best way to ensure that your doctor interprets your living will the way you want.

Be aware that living wills are invalid during pregnancy in many states. Still, if you want your wishes honored whether or not you're pregnant, write that in your living will. Doing so won't guarantee that your wishes are followed, but it will improve the chances.

States have different laws governing what information should go into a living will (see "State-specific considerations," page 25). While it's best to fill out a form clearly recognized by your state, our health decisions worksheet (page 35) or our generic living will (page 39) can help you think through important choices and serve as important documentation of your wishes.

Remember, it's not possible to know exactly how events will unfold when you become very ill or have a serious accident. Conversations and documents like a living will or the health decisions worksheet can help guide your health care agent and doctors in many situations, even those that you haven't directly discussed with them. Keep in mind, though, that living wills tend to be stuck in time. As your priorities and preferences change, a living will is harder to change than the health decisions worksheet or other less formal documents.

What is a do-not-resuscitate order (DNR)?

If you suffer cardiac arrest or stop breathing, people treating you are legally required to assume that you consent to cardiopulmonary resuscitation (CPR) to restore your breathing and heartbeat. This applies to both emergency medical technicians, who must resuscitate and stabilize you in order to bring you to the hospital, and to hospital personnel who treat you once you're there—unless you have a medical order that says otherwise, such as a do-not-resuscitate order (DNR) or physician orders for life-sustaining treatment (POLST; see next section).

Why would anyone want a DNR? If you have a terminal illness or little hope of improving enough to continue a life that's meaningful to you, you may wish to let nature take its course once your heart or breathing stops rather than having CPR. CPR is very often not successful and is physically traumatic (see "Understanding key medical procedures and programs," page 12). Before making this decision, however, discuss your situation with a doctor. A DNR order does not affect medical treatments other than CPR. Agreeing to a DNR, for example, does not affect whether you receive antibiotics or intravenous (IV) medications, so you will continue to receive the interventions that you want when you are sick.

There are reasons why you might *not* want a DNR, though. While DNRs were among the earliest documents that allowed a person to refuse a particular treatment (in this case, CPR), these forms are gradually being replaced with POLST, which is far more comprehensive. In a POLST form, CPR is just one of the options that you can accept or reject.

If you are caring for a terminally ill loved one, discuss how to handle an emergency before it happens. It may be that the first—or only—call your loved one will want you to make will be to hospice or the doctor for advice on comfort care. He or she may prefer this to calling 911, which would prompt a trip to the hospital and possibly unwanted and traumatic treatment if there is no DNR or if the ambulance and hospital staff don't have access to it.

Your primary care doctor can write a "non-hospital DNR" (also called an "out-of-hospital DNR") for emergency situations outside the hospital. Inside a hospital, the attending physician will need to translate your DNR into an in-hospital medical order for hospital staff to follow.

What are physician orders for life-sustaining treatment (POLST)?

If you are seriously ill right now, how can you help ensure that your goals and wishes for treatment will be honored if you are unable to speak for yourself when a medical emergency arises? Whether you want every medical option under the sun or simply want to be made comfortable (or something in between), POLST may be a helpful solution. In some states, POLST may go by the acronym POST (physician or provider orders for scope of treatment), MOLST (medical orders for life-sustaining treatment), or MOST (medical orders for scope of treatment). Regardless of the name, the approach is the same.

Developed in Oregon in 1991, POLST gives your wishes the authority of a medical order, signed by a physician or other authorized health care provider. This order should be based on a full discussion between you and the health care team about your condition and goals of care and what treatment options best suit your goals. Your health care agent can speak for you if you are too sick to participate. Following are some of the topics you and your doctor should discuss:

- Do you want comfort care only (for example, pain relief, wound care, and oxygen if needed to keep you comfortable)?
- Do you want comfort care plus limited additional treatments (for example, antibiotics or IV fluids)?
- Do you want full medical treatment (for example, mechanical ventilation and a variety of medications)?
- Do you want short-term or long-term artificial nutrition or no artificial nutrition at all?
- Do you want CPR if your heart or breathing stops?
- Do you want to avoid hospitalization (unless needed for comfort measures)?

POLST forms spell out these goals, and they do this using concrete orders that enable first responders and physicians to take action in emergencies. In this way, they are different from advance directives such as living wills. POLST orders reflect the care you want right now—if you had a medical crisis today—rather than care you might need in the distant future. By comparison, living wills provide more generalized treatment guidance and are not normally consulted in emergencies, when decisions must be made quickly. In emergency situations, first responders follow standard protocols unless medical orders such as POLST exist.

POLST is portable and effective across care settings. Thus, your wishes can guide treatment not only in an emergency, but also when you are in the hospital, at a nursing facility, or at home. The orders complement, but do not replace, any additional instructions offered in an advance directive or by your health care agent.

According to the National POLST Paradigm Task Force, this type of document is most appropriate for people who have serious, life-limiting conditions, which may include advanced frailty—in particular, people who are at risk of dying within the next year or two.

After your doctor completes and signs your POLST, he or she can, in many cases, place it in an electronic medical record for easy access by hospitals and other facilities where you get care. You should also post a copy at home where emergency medical personnel can see it (usually on the refrigerator), and carry one with you wherever you go. As with similar documents, you should revise your POLST when your circumstances or wishes change (see "Changing your advance care plan," page 26).

At this writing, 24 states have POLST programs that meet national standards, and 22 other states are developing them. Check with your doctor to learn if a POLST is appropriate for you and available where you live (see page 43 for a sample form).

Which advance directives do you need?

It's tempting to think that only elderly or very ill people need advance directives, but that's not the case. A serious accident or injury could result in decades of life without decision-making ability. But where do you start? Which documents do you really need? The following are some basic guidelines. (Because the differences between the various types of documents can be confusing, you may also want to refer to Table 1, page 7, for a summary of key features for each one.)

- Ideally, everyone should fill out a health care power of attorney to appoint a health care agent. Make this form your priority if you choose to have only one document. Appointing a health care agent you trust ensures that someone can act on your behalf for all medical decisions, not just the limited circumstances covered in a living will.
- You can also combine a power of attorney and living will. Be aware, however, that some experts believe a legally binding living will may actually limit your agent's power in ways that are not in your best interest (see "How specific should you be in your directives?" on page 11). Therefore, many experts recommend having a health care agent only and communicating your wishes in ways other than a formal living will, such as the health decisions worksheet (see Form 2, page 35).
- If you don't have anyone you trust to serve as your health care agent, you may want to have a living will.
- If you have a terminal disease or are suffering from advanced illness, you may also want to have a DNR or a POLST form, depending on which forms are permitted in your state (see "What is a do-not-resuscitate order (DNR)?" on page 5). Ask your doctor about these forms (and see page 43 for a sample POLST form). ▼

Table 1: Tools for advance care planning

FORM	DESCRIPTION	IS IT BINDING?	DOCUMENTS THAT TAKE PRECEDENCE	NOTES
▶ **Decision-making tools**				
Health decisions worksheet (see form, page 35)	This informal document, created for this publication, permits you to describe your wishes for care if you can't communicate them verbally. It also serves as a basis for discussion with your doctor, your family, and your health care agent.	No, it is not recognized as a legally valid advance directive, but it can help your health care agent and others better understand your values, care goals, and priorities.	Health care power of attorney, living will, and POLST (or equivalent) forms take legal precedence.	Make it clear to your agent that your wishes are to be treated as guidance, not binding instructions. You can transfer the information to a living will form, too.
Online tools (The Conversation Project, Five Wishes, others; see page 9)	Like the worksheet (previous entry), these tools take you through a process for determining, recording, and communicating your wishes for care.	No, these are not recognized as legally valid advance directives.	Health care power of attorney, living will, and POLST (or equivalent) forms take legal precedence.	Make it clear to your agent that your wishes are to be treated as guidance, not binding instructions. You can transfer the information to a living will form, too.
▶ **Legal tools**				
Health care power of attorney (see form, page 30)	This form allows you to name a person (called a health care agent or health care proxy) to make health care decisions for you if you are unable to do so yourself. It also allows you to name one or more alternate agents in case your first agent is unavailable or unwilling to serve.	Yes, it is legally recognized by statute in every state.	As long as you are able to make and communicate decisions, your word overrides anything you've written or told others. Only when you're unconscious or no longer have the capacity to make your wishes known does any advance directive swing fully into effect. Your agent is required to respect your goals and priorities for treatment, as you've described them.	If you complete only one advance directive, it should be this one. It is important to follow the legal requirements in your state for completing the document.
Living will (see form, page 39)	This legal document enables you to express your wishes about the kinds of medical care you would like to receive, or would like to avoid, if, at some point in the future, you are unable to communicate your wishes directly because of illness or incapacitation.	Yes, it is legally recognized by statute or practice in every state. Living will forms vary from state to state. Although a state may legally be required to honor any advance directive that clearly declares your wishes, it's best to fill out a form that your state recognizes.	Your oral statements take precedence over the living will, as long as you are able to make and communicate your decisions. You can state that the instructions given in your living will are intended as guidance, and your agent has the authority to interpret or modify your instructions in order to carry out what he or she believes are your values and wishes.	A living will is typically created well in advance of having a debilitating illness. At this writing, all states and the District of Columbia permit an advance directive that combines a living will with the appointment of a health care agent.
▶ **Medical orders**				
POLST (see sample form, page 43)	This is a medical order signed by a doctor or other health care professional after discussion about your care goals and priorities. It also requires your consent or that of your authorized representative.	Yes. Most states have adopted or are adopting a version of POLST.	POLST complements but does not replace any additional instructions given in a living will or by your health care agent. If your medical condition improves enough for you to make and express your decisions, your oral statements will again take precedence.	If you already have a serious, life-limiting medical condition, POLST is an important complement to other advance planning documents.
Do-not-resuscitate order (see page 5)	The out-of-hospital DNR is a medical order, signed by you and your physician, reflecting your wishes that emergency medical personnel not perform CPR if your heart or breathing stops.	Yes. However, to be effective in the hospital setting, your attending physician needs to translate your out-of-hospital DNR into an in-hospital DNR after a discussion with you or your surrogate. You do not need to sign this document.	You can revoke your consent to a DNR order at any time you are still able to make and communicate your decision. However, a hospital is not obligated to attempt resuscitation if it's clearly inappropriate.	POLST, which includes CPR as one option that can be accepted or rejected, is gradually replacing the non-hospital DNR in states that recognize POLST.

STEP 1 | Deciding on your wishes for care

Gathering information is the first step in deciding on your wishes for care. You can start by reading this chapter and talking to your doctor, if possible. In this chapter, we explain common medical procedures used when an emergency crops up—such as when your heart stops beating or you stop breathing—and we define important terms.

Understanding your health status

The first step in advance care planning is simply gaining a realistic understanding of your current health status. You may be in generally good health, despite having several medical conditions such as high blood pressure or osteoarthritis. You may be doing well now but have a chronic, progressive, ultimately fatal illness such as Alzheimer's disease or metastatic colon cancer. You may be frail because of multiple interacting chronic conditions or one disease that has widespread effects on your daily activities and health. Or you may have a serious advanced illness, such as end-stage heart failure.

Knowing which of these scenarios best characterizes your current situation and how your health is likely to evolve over the next several years will probably affect what goals are most important to you. Many people who are in generally good health would favor life-prolonging therapy in the event of any new, acute medical problem such as pneumonia or a heart attack. Some people with progressive, chronic illness also favor life-prolonging therapy in the event of a new problem or worsening of their chronic condition; others regard their daily functioning as of paramount concern. Many people who are frail are primarily concerned with retaining their independence and maximizing their quality of life; because their frailty may become more severe with aggressive medical treatments, they may prefer to limit such treatment. Finally, people in the final stage of a serious illness—whether metastatic cancer, end-stage heart disease, or advanced Alzheimer's disease—often wish comfort to be the overriding aim of medical treatment. Accordingly, they would decline CPR, admission to an intensive care unit, surgery, or other invasive treatment in the event of an acute illness.

If you have a major medical condition, the best way to understand your prognosis is to talk to your doctor. Following are some useful questions to ask in gathering information:
- What is the usual course of this condition?
- What is known about it, and what is unknown?
- What are my chances of recovery?
- What will the "new normal" be after recovery?
- What are the chances that I'll be worse off?
- How will a (recommended) treatment affect my functioning?
- Are there other possible treatments?
- What side effects will I likely experience?
- What will life be like after this treatment?
- If pain or discomfort is involved, how will that be managed?

Prioritizing your goals for care

Once you have a clearer understanding of your health status, you need to decide upon your goals for care. This is the single most important step in the process, followed of course by communicating that information to your family and physician. The forms are merely a way of trying to capture those decisions and translate them into practical plans for care in the event of illness.

All of us have goals for care, stated or not. After an illness or injury, you may hope to return to your life feeling and acting the same as you did before. But that may not be possible. A brain injury, complications from diabetes or a heart ailment, or health issues related to aging can change your life in major and minor ways, sometimes within a matter of hours or even minutes.

Continued on page 10

Online tools

Several interactive websites can help guide you through the process of deciding on your wishes and communicating those to others. Some of them also take you through the steps to complete a formal advance directive. Here are some options to explore.

Advance Planning for Dementia. This free planning tool can help you think through what kind of care you would want to receive if you had mild, moderate, or severe dementia. You can download this document, fill it out, and share it with your health care agent and your doctor. For more information, see https://dementia-directive.org.

The Conversation Project. Founded in 2010 by newspaper columnist Ellen Goodman and like-minded colleagues, The Conversation Project focuses on helping people talk to loved ones and doctors about desires for end-of-life care. The multimedia website offers a mix of how-to advice and thought-provoking personal stories and quotes from a wide range of people who've embarked on these conversations. A free starter kit is available in English and Spanish. It uses prompts to help you collect your thoughts on the role you prefer to play in health decisions, where you'd like to be cared for, and what sort of care you want. The website also offers ways to kick-start and guide an end-of-life conversation, and a questionnaire designed to help you talk to your doctor. For more information, see www.theconversationproject.org.

Five Wishes. Written very simply, Five Wishes is an advance directive that helps you clarify and convey your personal, spiritual, and emotional wishes as well as medical ones. It was developed in Florida in 1997 through the nonprofit organization Aging with Dignity and currently meets the legal requirements for advance directives in most states. For $5 (at this writing), Five Wishes can be filled out online in English or by hand on a paper form,

available in 26 languages. The form encourages you to answer five direct end-of-life questions:

- Whom do you choose to make decisions on your behalf?
- Which medical treatments do you want or not want?
- How comfortable do you want to be made?
- How do you want people to treat you?
- What do you want loved ones to know?

For more information, see www.fivewishes.org.

Go Wish. This is a game you play either for free online or with a pack of special cards that list priorities you may have for your care near the end of life. Examples include "Not being connected to machines," "To be free from pain," and "To have close friends near." As you play it, you sort through what's most important to you and put the cards into piles titled "very important," "somewhat important," and "not important." You can also play it with your health care agent. Developed by Coda Alliance, a nonprofit organization, the cards are available in English and Spanish through the Go Wish website for $26 per pack (at this writing). The website also links to other sites where you can buy the cards in several other languages. For more information, see www.gowish.org.

MyDirectives. This online tool uses an interactive decision program to enable you to create a document that combines a living will and a health care power of attorney. This document can be accessed by your health care providers. You also can express your preferences about resuscitation, organ donation, and autopsy. The tool makes it possible to give detailed answers and even include audio or video file attachments and emergency contact information. There's also an app version for iPhone. MyDirectives is operated by

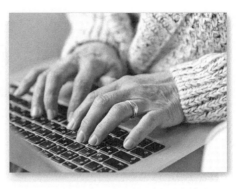

a for-profit company, ADVault, Inc., but the service is free to individuals. Health care and health insurance providers pay fees to access it. For more information, see https://mydirectives.com.

Prepare for Your Care. Available in English or Spanish, the website of this nonprofit organization takes you through a free, step-by-step process to think through your needs and preferences about end-of-life care. You can save your answers in a document called "Summary of My Wishes." You also can fill out an advance directive form online, or you can download and print either document. The site also includes videos about people facing health decisions. Their examples are intended to help you

- choose a medical decision maker
- decide what matters most in life
- choose how much flexibility you want your decision maker to have
- tell others about your wishes
- ask doctors the right questions.

Prepare for Your Care is based on the research of Dr. Rebecca Sudore, a professor of medicine at the University of California, San Francisco. She found that people using the website were more likely to fill out an advance directive form than those who were given the form alone. For more information, see https://prepareforyourcare.org.

Other approaches

Other comprehensive approaches to advance care planning, such as Respecting Choices and the ACP Decisions video series, may be available through your doctor or hospital.

Continued from page 8

Usually, people have three goals of care related to illness or injury:

- prolonging life
- obtaining maximum comfort (such as pain relief)
- maintaining daily function.

If, at a given stage of life, all three of these goals can't be met, you must determine which goal is of most importance to you. From there, you can identify what types of interventions are consistent with your stated priorities.

One common goal is recovering from an illness or injury sufficiently to return to activities that make life meaningful to you. If this is your goal, you need to offer guidance on what is—and isn't—meaningful life. Some people say, "As long as I can open my eyes, sit up, and recognize my family, that's all I want. I don't care if I have to be fed and bathed and have my bottom wiped by someone else." In that scenario, health care providers will make the decisions needed to make sure those goals are achieved. Someone else might say, "You know what? If I can't read a book and talk about it with my family, if I can't feed myself and toilet myself, and my condition is only going to get worse, I don't want to be alive."

When recovery isn't possible—if you have an incurable cancer, for example, or your body is winding down from a combination of illnesses accumulated over time—your goal may shift to comfort care, which focuses on easing pain and other distressing symptoms, rather than a cure, so that you are better able to enjoy the time you have left.

Because the goals of care usually change as your medical situation changes, advance care planning is an ongoing process.

Talking to your doctor about treatment options

Even the most fertile imagination can't cover all the possibilities for care during an emergency or toward the end of life. And sometimes trying to be very specific—saying "do everything possible to bring me back" or "don't ever tube-feed me"—can backfire. You may not understand what a medical term truly means, or the option you dismiss might just be the bridge you need

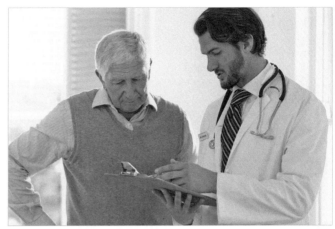

It helps to speak with a doctor before you finalize your wishes for care in a document. A doctor can explain medical terms and discuss with you what's likely or unlikely to work in your situation.

to reach partial or full recovery. A doctor can explain medical terms and discuss what's possible and what isn't likely to work given your specific health issues and goals of care. Further, a doctor can help you consider circumstances under which you might decide to have, or decide to forgo, such treatments or procedures as CPR, artificial nutrition, hydration, and hemodialysis (see "Understanding key medical procedures and programs," page 12). For all of these reasons, it helps to talk to a doctor before you finalize your wishes for care in a document or through conversations with your health care agent, family, and close friends.

It's equally important to make sure your doctor is willing to follow your directive. (This assumes you have a regular personal physician. If not, it is important to choose one.) If a doctor disagrees with your wishes, he or she does not have to carry them out, but is obligated to attempt to find a doctor who will. To avoid this complication, make sure your doctor is comfortable with your decisions. Schedule an appointment with him or her specifically to go over your completed advance directive.

During the conversation, tell your doctor how much you would like to know about your condition should you become very ill. Some people want to know everything, some prefer only the basics, and some want their family members to receive the information and make decisions for them. Note how much information you want shared with your loved ones. If you wish, you can exclude particular persons from

Standard emergency care: What does it entail?

Standard care for emergencies is more far-reaching than many people realize. These questions and answers address what steps medical staff may take if you are seriously ill and you haven't declined any specific procedures in advance.

What is "standard care" in an emergency?

If your heart stops beating and you stop breathing, the first step is cardiopulmonary resuscitation (CPR)—a combination of chest compressions, artificial respiration, and defibrillation to shock the heart back into a steady rhythm.

What if basic CPR is not sufficient?

Sometimes your heart will start beating using basic CPR, but often the heart needs more than just a quick restart to continue working—for example, you may need repeated defibrillator shocks or even a temporary pacemaker. Moreover, you may still not able to breathe independently. That's when doctors move on to advanced cardiac life support. You would be intubated—that is, a tube is inserted through the nose, mouth, or throat into the trachea. The tube would be attached to a breathing machine called a ventilator or respirator that pushes air into and out of the lungs. Intravenous medications to raise or lower blood pressure, control heart rate, or make the kidneys work better might be given.

If you were in a hospital, the staff would draw blood to check how well your lungs, kidneys, and liver are working, find out if you have an infection, and make sure you have enough essential minerals in your blood. A catheter would be placed in your bladder to drain urine. If your kidneys weren't working properly, you might have dialysis. Imaging scans, other tests, and, if necessary, surgery would be done as well.

That's pretty extensive. Wouldn't these be considered "heroic measures"?

Such measures may seem extreme or heroic, but they are the standard of care in the United States in order to save a life. If you want anything less done, you have to be explicit.

What if I say, yes, please do CPR, but no, don't put me on a ventilator?

You could say that. But if you're so sick that your heart stopped beating and you stopped breathing, it's unlikely that your doctor would be able to bring you back by just pushing on your chest and shocking your heart. Usually, if the heart stops, the lungs stop breathing, too. Mouth-to-mouth respiration can provide oxygen for a few minutes, but beyond that you need the ventilator. To decide that you only want part of the intervention doesn't really make sense.

How should I discuss this with my doctor?

The first step is to begin the conversation. You can start by telling your doctor that you have been reading about this and would like to discuss resuscitation—what it is, what it would mean for you given your medical problems, and whether you would want to receive it.

---

having any role in decisions by saying so or writing it into your advance directive.

Once you've filled out an advance directive, ask your doctor to scan the form into your electronic medical record (or copy it for a paper medical file) and add relevant notes about your conversations on these topics. If you have a change of heart or circumstances, update your directive as appropriate with your doctor (see "Changing your advance care plan," page 26). Periodically, check that your doctor has current contact information for your health care agent.

How specific should you be in your directives?

A good rule to follow is this: the closer you are to decisions that are likely to arise because of known health problems, the more specific you can be in your instruc-tions. For example, if you have very strong wishes about treatments you know you are likely to face because of your current medical condition, it makes sense to include these wishes in a formal living will.

Otherwise, it's best not to be too specific. Why? It's impossible to know all the medical facts and variables that will be important in a future decision.

For example, suppose you opt to appoint a health care agent and to fill out a living will. Let's say this liv-ing will states that under no circumstances do you want to be fed artificially—that is, through a tube or intravenously. Your agent may not be able to overrule these written instructions, even if you would need artificial nutrition only for a relatively short time to help you fully recover.

Furthermore, medicine advances rapidly. New tests, medications, and technologies arrive at a speed that outstrips our ability to see how these changes will affect our lives. You may not want to be locked into specific medical treatments that aren't optimal when the time arrives.

To avoid such a situation, there are two options. One is to appoint a health care agent (see Form 1, page 30) and fill out just the health decisions worksheet on page 35 rather than a formal living will. Doing so will help clarify your goals for care, without being legally binding. You can give a copy of this worksheet to your agent and change it easily as your preferences or circumstances change. Be sure to discuss your treatment goals and priorities with your agent. The second option is to complete a living will, but state clearly in the document that your instructions constitute guidance and are not mandatory. And, in your health care power of attorney, expressly state that you intend your agent's authority to interpret your wishes to be as broad as possible.

In addition, no matter which advance planning documents you use, try to give your agent as much guidance as you feel comfortable giving through conversations.

Understanding key medical procedures and programs

Following are explanations of common medical procedures that may be recommended during the course of a serious illness or at the end of life. As you read, think about whether you can foresee conditions under which you would, or would not, want certain procedures or care. Understanding these concepts will help as you fill out the health decisions worksheet. You needn't make these important decisions by yourself. We encourage you to talk to your doctor about your goals and get his or her recommendations about what care to seek given your state of health. Realize that the desirability of any these interventions may depend on your circumstances (see "Life-sustaining vs. organ-sustaining treatment," page 13).

Artificial nutrition

When you are unable to swallow anything by mouth, this procedure supplies nutrients and fluids through a nasogastric tube inserted through your nose into your stomach (a short-term approach), through a gastrostomy tube inserted directly through your abdominal wall into your stomach (a longer-term approach), or sometimes through a jejunostomy tube (similar to a gastrostomy tube, but inserted into the small intestine, also for a longer term). Or, if your gut isn't working properly, you could be given nutrients and fluids intravenously, through a central vein, such as the jugular. Called parenteral nutrition, this is another long-term strategy.

Artificial nutrition may be used as a bridge when the underlying problem is temporary and you are likely to recover. It may also be used long-term to help keep a person with an irreversible condition alive, although it will not necessarily improve quality of life. In certain conditions, such as advanced dementia, artificial nutrition is often used to improve quality of life or prolong life, but there is no evidence it does either. Inserting a gastrostomy tube is a surgical procedure, and because patients with dementia have a tendency to pull out the tube, they are sometimes physically restrained to prevent them from doing so. People who choose not to have artificial nutrition often do so because they wish to avoid the discomfort involved.

Intravenous (artificial) hydration

When a person is unable to swallow anything by mouth, artificial hydration supplies a solution of water, sugar, and minerals through an intravenous (IV) tube placed into a vein. If the problem is likely to be short-lived—say, a few days—hydration alone may be sufficient to provide necessary liquids and calories; otherwise, artificial nutrition must be considered as well.

Like artificial nutrition, hydration may be used temporarily when the person is likely to recover sufficiently to take fluids by mouth. Or it may be used long-term in the case of an irreversible condition to help keep a person alive, although it will not improve quality of life. People might choose not to have artificial hydration to avoid the discomfort involved or because they wish not to prolong the dying process.

Cardiopulmonary resuscitation (CPR)

If your heart and breathing stop and you become unconscious, CPR can be used to try to resuscitate you. A simple form of CPR—known as "bystander CPR," as it is designed to be performed by members of the public in an emergency before EMTs arrive—

Life-sustaining vs. organ-sustaining treatment

It's possible to keep a person alive—technically, anyway—long after essential sparks of life seem to have disappeared, says Dr. Muriel Gillick, the medical editor of this report. Here, Dr. Gillick answers some of the questions she grapples with in her work.

Q. Can you explain the terms "life-sustaining" and "organ-sustaining"?
A. Most of the medical treatments we talk about when we discuss life-sustaining treatment are intended to bolster a single organ whose function is profoundly impaired: artificial ventilation—that is, intubation and use of a respirator—is used to compensate for lung failure, CPR is used when the heart stops pumping, and dialysis makes up for the inability of the kidneys to cleanse the blood of waste products. So they are organ-sustaining treatments. But whether the treatments will simply support that organ or will actually help restore a person to something like the condition he or she was in before depends in part on whether the organ failure is just temporary and in part on how well the rest of the body is functioning.

Q. But organ-sustaining treatment is helpful in some circumstances, isn't it?
A. Absolutely! A respirator can be life-sustaining in patients with severe pneumonia, perhaps involving multiple lobes of the lung, who need help breathing until antibiotics and the body's immune system kick in to treat the pneumonia—but not in patients with very severe emphysema and no infection. CPR can save lives for patients who have a heart attack complicated by a very dangerous electrical disturbance in the heart called a ventricular arrhythmia, but are otherwise in good health—but not of patients who are dying from widely metastatic cancer. And dialysis can keep patients with end-stage kidney disease alive and able to function if the other organs, such as the heart and the brain, are all working normally—but not in patients in their 80s and 90s with other major chronic conditions. Many of these technologies were designed to be used short-term for readily reversible problems, but they are increasingly tried for irreversible problems or in patients with multiple other medical problems.

Q. How do you counsel patients to make use of these techniques?
A. I like to start by making sure patients understand their current state of health. If they realize they are very frail or have a progressive, life-threatening illness, I can explain that most "life-sustaining" technologies probably won't help. I also try to figure out the patient's goals for care. Once they've grappled with what's most important to them, I can help them decide if a given technology is likely to achieve their goals. I reassure them that deciding to forgo a burdensome treatment is not the same as committing suicide—it is simply balancing the risks and benefits of different approaches to care. Sometimes there's a great deal of uncertainty about how effective a particular treatment will be in a given clinical situation. In that case, I recommend a limited trial: letting the doctors try the treatment for a specified period of time and then re-evaluating whether to continue based on how the patient is responding to the treatment. Withdrawing treatment is not euthanasia, the deliberate ending of life by a physician; rather, it involves discontinuing an ineffective or excessively burdensome treatment.

---

is taught by the American Heart Association. This technique focuses on hard, fast chest compressions at a rate of 100 to 120 times per minute. As a guide to reaching that speed, the association tells people to think of the beat of the disco song "Stayin' Alive."

When hospital personnel or emergency medical technicians (EMTs) perform CPR, they use three combined techniques.

- Artificial respiration employs a plastic mask placed over the mouth and nose. The mask is attached to a tube and bag. The bag is squeezed and released, moving air in and out of the lungs of a person who has stopped breathing.

- Artificial circulation entails repeatedly pressing on the chest (chest compressions) to squeeze blood out of a heart that no longer is pumping.

- Defibrillation involves using a medical device called a defibrillator that delivers an electric shock to the body to reset an abnormal heart rhythm to a normal, steady rhythm.

In movies and TV dramas, CPR seems to be astoundingly successful. The reality is less rosy: for someone given CPR in the hospital, the overall rate of survival to discharge is less than 25%. Survival rates are even lower for frail, older individuals or for anyone who receives CPR outside a hospital—although the widespread availability of automated external defibrillators (AEDs) has allowed some bystanders to resuscitate people without full CPR. In fact, an AED can nearly double the chances of survival if someone suffers cardiac arrest outside of a hospital. (Essentially, all you have to do is push a button. AEDs

Organ donation

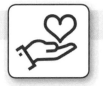

As you're thinking about care in the last stages of life, one thing to consider is whether you would want to become an organ donor if circumstances allow at the time of your death.

Health care providers work hard to save every patient's life. But sometimes there is a complete and irreversible loss of brain function, or blood flow and breathing. In these circumstances, the person is declared clinically and legally dead according to accepted medical standards. Only then is donation an option.

People of all ages and medical histories are potential organ and tissue donors. The feasibility of organ or tissue donation is evaluated at the time of death, and even advanced age is not a deal breaker. More than 100,000 people are waiting for lifesaving transplants every day, so the need for organ and tissue donors always remains critical. Besides major organs, a wide range of other tissues may be transplantable. They include corneas, heart valves, bone, tendons, skin, and blood.

There is no cost to the donor's family or estate for organ donation. The donor's family members pay only for medical expenses before death and for funeral costs, as they would in any case. Funeral arrangements can continue as planned after organ donation occurs.

If you would like your organs to be considered for donation, it's important to make these wishes known. You can include an organ donation consent and instructions in your advance directive or in a separate organ donor form. In many states, you also can put a notation of your consent on your driver's license. In addition, it helps to enter your name in your state's organ donor registry, because that is often the first place the hospital will check. To sign up, simply go to www.organdonor.gov. Be sure to tell your health care agent and other close family members about your decision.

It is important to appreciate that, for potential donors, certain medical interventions are necessary after death to keep the organs viable for donation. These could include injection of certain medications and possible use of a ventilator to temporarily continue blood supply and oxygen to the organs.

are now available for use by laypersons in airports, shopping malls, schools, and other public venues. A person's body jerks when the shock is delivered, but recipients of defibrillation are usually unconscious and won't remember it, although they may feel sore and achy afterward.)

The success of CPR, however, depends on a variety of medical circumstances, including what kind of illness the person has, how severe it is, and how long after cardiac arrest CPR is started. When someone has a terminal illness, the odds of revival are extremely low. Moreover, CPR can injure the body. For example, bruising on the chest is common, and ribs sometimes get broken in the process. In contrast, death from cardiac arrest is sudden and mostly pain-

free. Some people who are sick or dying decide to forgo CPR because they simply feel it's "too much."

Intubation and mechanical ventilation

If the combined techniques of CPR should fail, the next step is advanced cardiac life support, including intubation and mechanical ventilation, plus drugs to stimulate a stopped or failing heart.

A machine called a ventilator or respirator (sometimes called a breathing machine) pushes air into the lungs, replacing or supporting the lungs' normal function when a person cannot breathe unassisted. Patients on a breathing machine may be conscious or unconscious. A tube attached to the machine is inserted into the nose, mouth, or throat and passed down into the trachea (windpipe). This is called intubation. To relieve the discomfort of the tube in the windpipe, physicians often administer sedatives. When the breathing tube is inserted through the nose or mouth, a person cannot talk.

Mechanical ventilation can be used short-term as a bridge to recovery, or over a longer period. People on mechanical ventilation for longer than a week also need other organ-sustaining treatments, including artificial nutrition and a catheter to remove waste from the bladder. They move their bowels into a bedpan. Bedsores may develop. If a person becomes well enough to stop using the ventilator, physical therapy is typically necessary, often in a rehabilitation center, to help get the person back on his or her feet after a period of prolonged bed rest. If the breathing tube needs to be used for more than two to three weeks, it will be moved from the nose or mouth and inserted into the windpipe through a surgical incision in the front of the neck (a tracheostomy).

When a person is terminally ill, mechanical ventilation may prolong the dying process, but it cannot treat the underlying condition or improve quality of life. People who choose not to be placed on mechanical ventilators might make that decision for any of several reasons, including not wanting to be sedated or unable to talk. Some people don't want their families to see them tied to machines in an incoherent state or do not want to spend what may be their last days in a hospital bed.

In deciding whether or not to accept intubation, you should know that a less invasive alternative is now available that may be effective, depending on the clinical situation. Bilevel positive airway pressure (BiPAP) is an adaptation of the more familiar continuous positive airway pressure (CPAP) device sometimes used in people with sleep apnea (episodes of not breathing during sleep). BiPAP masks, which are held in place by straps, might cover the full face, the nose area, the mouth area, or both the nose and mouth. The availability of noninvasive ventilation also means that you may be asked to decide not just whether you would accept a ventilator, but also whether you would be willing to undergo treatment with BiPAP or a related device.

Hemodialysis

When you're well, your kidneys maintain the right balance of fluids and essential minerals (sodium, potassium, calcium, and others) in your body, and clear wastes from your blood. If your kidneys fail temporarily or permanently, a dialysis machine can mimic these tasks by filtering your blood. Typically, needles are placed in two sites in your arm so blood flows through one tube into the machine to be filtered, then is pumped back into your arm through the second tube. The treatment (typically referred to simply as dialysis) usually requires three weekly sessions, each of which takes three to five hours, at home or at a clinic.

Depending on your overall life situation, you may wish to pursue this treatment, or you may decide

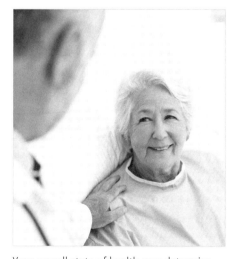

Your overall state of health may determine whether or not a treatment like dialysis is worth the time and discomfort.

to forgo it. For instance, if you are generally healthy but your kidneys are failing, you may feel dialysis is worth the effort. People often feel better when their blood has been purged of waste products, although only on days when they are not receiving dialysis. In contrast, if you are old and frail and you have several other chronic health problems, dialysis is unlikely to prolong your life, and you may decide the discomfort of the procedure is not worth the effort. Over all, whether the benefits outweigh the burdens is a highly individual decision. People who choose not to have hemodialysis might do so because of the physical exhaustion, discomfort, and time involved, particularly if other health issues compromise their ability to lead a meaningful life.

Palliative care

Palliative care is supportive care for people with serious advanced illnesses and their family members. It aims to keep a patient comfortable and pain-free by using a combination of evidence-based measures to treat distressing symptoms. Hospice (see below) is one means of offering this type of care, but palliative care is far more comprehensive: in addition to symptom relief, it also addresses psychological issues (such as depression), family conflict, caregiver stress, and advance care planning. It is recommended for people with serious illnesses before the end stage of their disease, and—unlike hospice—it can be given concurrently with life-prolonging care.

Palliative care is available in most hospitals. You or your family can request a consultation with a palliative care specialist through your attending physician. Such services are also increasingly available to non-hospitalized patients through a community-based, interdisciplinary team approach. You can request these services through your primary care doctor.

Hospice

When curative treatments can no longer help or when further treatment seems futile, many people

© Neustockimages | Getty Images

focus instead on comfort care for troubling symptoms like pain or difficulty breathing. Hospice, a medical benefit covered by Medicare and most other health insurance providers, is a program of care designed to deliver this. In 2016, 1.4 million Americans received hospice services through Medicare, according to the National Hospice and Palliative Care Organization. More than one million people who died in the United States were under the care of a hospice program.

Hospice takes a team approach to care, drawing together the skills of a doctor, nurse, home health aide, social worker, spiritual counselor, and volunteers. You need a doctor's referral to hospice, stipulating that you have been diagnosed with an incurable condition and are likely to die within six months. Death doesn't always occur within that time frame, of course, and some people stay with hospice for much longer. It's worth noting that your doctor may suggest hospice long before you are actively dying. Entering a hospice program need not signal "giving up"; rather, you and your loved ones may welcome the extra support and compassionate care that hospice provides.

Most hospice care (57%) is given in the place a person calls home—a private residence, an assisted living facility, or a nursing home, according to the National Hospice and Palliative Care Organization. Alternatively, you may move to a hospice facility if one is available, or receive hospice services at a hospital. The hospice team responds to the wide-ranging needs of the dying person, family, and caregivers. Hospice may deliver such helpful supplies or equipment as a hospital bed, oxygen, or medications to help quell pain, anxiety, or infections that interfere with breathing. Usually, grief counseling is offered for family members and caregivers for 13 months following a death.

Organ-sustaining treatment

A set of drugs, medical procedures, and machines that may keep a person alive for an indefinite period of time, but which cannot cure a terminal condition, is collectively known as organ-sustaining treatment. A few examples are hemodialysis (see page 15), mechanical ventilation (see page 14), and artificial nutrition (see page 12).

Often this is called "life-sustaining" treatment, although some experts argue that "organ-sustaining" treatment is a more appropriate description (see "Life-sustaining vs. organ-sustaining treatment," page 13). While such treatments can serve as an important bridge to recovery, sometimes they merely postpone death without supporting meaningful life.

Medical terms to know

When preparing an advance directive, it's helpful to have an understanding of a handful of medical terms often heard in end-of-life discussions. Refer back to this list as you fill out the forms in this report.

Brain death. This means that electrical activity in the entire brain is absent. Pupils are fixed and dilated. The heart continues to beat, but the person lies in an irreversible state of unconsciousness without reflexes, deliberate movements, or the ability to breathe without mechanical ventilation.

Coma. A person in a coma is in a deep sleeplike state of unconsciousness from which he or she cannot be wakened. The eyes remain closed, and the person exhibits no emotion and no response to noise or painful stimulation. A coma may be reversible, may progress to a vegetative state, or may resolve but leave a person with profound disabilities.

Minimally conscious state. A person is considered minimally conscious if he or she shows occasional moments of awareness, such as smiling or crying in response to emotional stimuli, vocalizing, reaching for objects, or tracking with the eyes. A minority of people emerge from a minimally conscious state, but when they do, they often have major disabilities.

Vegetative state. A person in a vegetative state appears to be awake, with open eyes. He or she may yawn, cough, or make occasional movements, but exhibits few meaningful responses to the environment. The brainstem is working, so the person is still breathing and the heart is still beating, but other brain functions such as thought, speech, and purposeful movement have ceased. After a person has been in a vegetative state for a month or more, he or she is considered to be in a persistent vegetative state, which is irreversible. ◆

STEP 2 Choosing a health care agent

Selecting an effective health care agent requires thought. Though you may reflexively turn to your spouse or oldest child, he or she may not necessarily be the best person to fulfill this role. Other family members or friends might be better choices. And in some cases, you may have to look beyond those options. In choosing a health care agent, you also need to be aware of state-specific laws that may eliminate certain people from consideration. In this chapter, we explain the basics, then offer suggestions for broaching tough topics as well as tips you can share to help your health care agent handle the task.

The basics

Here arc some fundamental questions and answers to consider when choosing a health care agent.

What does the law say?

Legal requirements whittle down some choices right away. In most states, certain people cannot be your health care agent, including your attending physician and, in some states, any health care worker in your medical facility or nursing home. In most states, people must be 18 or older to serve as an agent. Some states won't allow you to appoint a person who is serving as the agent for 10 or more people, unless he or she is your spouse or close relative.

You can view your state-specific restrictions on health care agents online at www.health.harvard.edu/state-limits.

Whom should you choose?

You can rule people out—or in—by answering a few questions about each of them:

- Do you trust this person to make life-and-death decisions for you?
- Does this person understand your wishes and feel comfortable going along with them?
- Does this person live close enough to be with you easily? It's possible to handle the duties of a health care agent by phone, but it helps to be available in person.
- Will this person be too emotionally involved to make important decisions? For example, it may seem logical to appoint your daughter because you feel very close to her. But will she have trouble carrying out certain wishes—for instance, if you decide

▶ Looking beyond friends and family

What if you have no trusted friend or family member to act as your health care agent? You'd be wise to consider other options. If you are part of a religious community, for example, you might ask another congregant or a religious leader to consider being your health care agent. Alternatively, you might ask your lawyer.

In the future, you might also have the option of appointing a "health fiduciary"—a new type of professional who is trained and certified to act as a surrogate decision maker for people who are unable to make decisions for themselves. But at present, if there is absolutely no one appropriate to serve as your agent, then a living will is your best fallback tool.

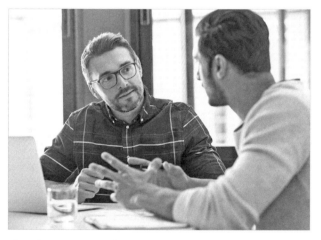

If you have no trusted friend or family member to serve as your health care agent, consider asking your lawyer or religious leader.

© shapecharge | Getty Images

you want dialysis stopped if you aren't improving, or that you don't wish to have CPR?

- Can this person manage potential conflict among family members?
- Will this person question health care providers in order to fully understand your medical condition and treatment options?
- Is this person able and willing to be persistent with your doctors and stand up for your wishes?

Can you appoint more than one agent?

Many states require you to authorize just one agent at a time. Even if that's not the case, appointing more than one can complicate matters because any disagreement among your agents would pose a serious barrier. If you are a parent, you may not feel comfortable choosing one adult child over another, but if you talk this through with your children, you may find that one is more willing or better suited to take on this role.

You can instruct your agent to consult with someone else. For example, if you want to appoint your daughter because you know she could strongly advocate for your wishes, but you feel your son would be helpful in making some decisions, you can ask your daughter to seek advice from him to the extent practical. Legally, though, she would still be the only person responsible for making decisions.

If possible, appoint an alternate agent in case your first choice is unwilling to act or unavailable when needed. Naming a second alternate is a good idea as well if you have more than one person you would trust in that role.

Commonly held myths about end-of-life issues

Myth: Refusing life support invalidates your life insurance, because you are committing suicide.
Truth: Refusing life support does not mean that you are committing suicide. Rather, the underlying medical problem would be considered to be the cause of death.

Myth: If medical treatment is started, it cannot be stopped.
Truth: Not starting a medical treatment and stopping a treatment are the same in the eyes of the law, so you or your health care agent can approve a potentially helpful treatment for a trial period without fear that you can't change your mind later. However, be aware that stopping treatment can be more difficult emotionally than not starting it in the first place.

Myth: If you refuse organ-sustaining treatments, you're refusing all treatments.
Truth: No matter what treatments you refuse, you will still receive any other care you need or want—both pain and symptom management and curative care.

Myth: It's painful to stop or refuse artificial nutrition and hydration.
Truth: Unlike keeping food or water from a healthy person, declining artificial nutrition or intravenous hydration does not cause pain in most critically ill individuals.

Myth: More care is always better.
Truth: Not necessarily. Two decades of research from the Dartmouth Atlas Project underscore problems with this line of thought. The researchers found that, in regions that deliver a higher volume of care, Medicare patients go into the hospital more frequently, clock more time in intensive care units, visit doctors more often, and receive more diagnostic tests than matched peers in regions where less medical care is the norm. That translates to higher health care costs, but not better health outcomes or improved survival rates after heart attacks or hip fractures.

Can your power of attorney for financial matters make medical decisions for you?

No. Usually, the person you name as having power of attorney can only make financial decisions for you. You need to appoint a health care agent to make medical decisions. However, you can select the same individual to perform both tasks for you if you so desire.

What happens if you don't choose an agent or fill out a living will?

If you lose the ability to make your own decisions, most states permit a close relative or friend to do so. However, this may not be the person you would prefer to make decisions for you. Typically, state laws provide a hierarchy of authorized decision makers, starting with one's spouse, followed by an adult child, parent, and sibling, down through some degree of relationship. About half of the states include a close friend as decision maker where there is no authorized family member available.

In a medical emergency, treatment decisions may fall to the attending doctor. However, it's better not to let that happen. A study published in *Annals of Internal Medicine* looked at more than 3,000 critically ill patients in seven medical centers throughout the United States. About one in 20 deaths occurred in people without a surrogate decision maker. In those cases, physicians faced with the same clinical circumstances made widely differing decisions regarding life support. These variations seemed to be related to the physician's personal preferences as much as to the patient's wishes and his or her illness.

If it is not an emergency, and no close relative or friend can help, a court might have to appoint a guardian—a person or a government agency—to make medical and other decisions for you. This can take time, which may affect your care. And, of course, the person or people appointed by a judge as decision makers may or may not know you and your wishes.

Guardianship is a drastic move, and having a health care power of attorney will normally avoid the need for guardianship, unless something goes wrong—for example, your agent acts inappropriately or other conflicts arise that cannot be worked out. Even if a guardian is appointed, most states continue to recognize your agent unless the court revokes your agent's authority. If you have documented your wishes in an advance directive, normally a guardian must follow your known wishes.

Talking to your health care agent

Before you appoint someone as your health care agent (or alternate agent), you'll have to make sure that person understands your wishes and is willing to carry them out. If he or she objects to one of your decisions, you might want to pick someone else. Try these tips for broaching the subject with your agent:

Do your homework. Filling out the health decisions worksheet on page 35 will give you a good sense of what you want to say. It may help to include any religious beliefs that influence your thoughts on end-

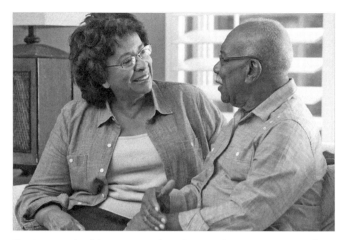

Serving as a health care agent is an honor—it means someone literally trusts you with his or her life—but first, have a conversation to make sure you feel comfortable carrying out the person's wishes.

of-life issues, and your goals and priorities for medical care, if you've decided on these.

Lead with an easy opening. When you first raise the subject with the person you'd like to be your agent, you might try something like this: "I just filled out this health decisions worksheet, which explains what I'd like done if I become very ill. It says that I should talk about my wishes with someone I trust and appoint him or her to make decisions for me if I'm not able to. I'd like to talk to you about this." If the person is uncomfortable, be persistent and explain how important it is to you. If he or she refuses to discuss it, choose another agent.

Focus on everyone's well-being. If you're nervous about discussing end-of-life care with your agent, remember that the conversation will make his or her job easier. Being responsible for making medical choices for someone you care about is difficult, and any uncertainty makes it even harder. Talking about options for care that matter to you and putting those choices in writing are as important to peace of mind for your family and friends as to you.

Set the scene. If you are having trouble broaching the topic, it may be helpful to refer to a recent TV show, movie, or news broadcast that touched on end-of-life care. Some people find it helps to reminisce about people who have passed away. Others appreciate having their doctor, religious adviser, or a close friend mediate the conversation.

Share with others. Sharing your wishes with a

wider circle of family and friends may give your agent more support—as well as oversight—since more than one person will know what you've decided. You can let these people know that you've prepared an advance directive, and then say something like, "I'd feel better knowing that you were aware of my wishes. Can we talk about this?" Such a discussion also serves to prevent later objections to decisions your agent may make on your behalf, since they won't be a surprise.

Tips for being an effective health care agent

Being asked to be someone's health care agent is a special honor—it means the person is saying, "I trust you with my life." That said, it's also a huge responsibility. Before you say yes, make sure that you feel comfortable carrying out the person's wishes and that you don't feel morally or religiously opposed to their requests. Once you have agreed to be someone's agent, the following tips may help you do a better job:

- Realize that your legal and ethical duty as agent is to make decisions in keeping with your loved one's instructions, if any, and other values, goals, and priorities to the extent that you know them. Otherwise, you must make decisions that are in the person's best interest, taking into account his or her values, to the extent that you know them.

- Be sure you know everything possible about your loved one's values, goals, and priorities at the time the health care power of attorney is signed. And check in with him or her every now and then—especially after a change in health—to find out if those feelings have changed.

- If your loved one becomes sick, be sure the staff of the nursing home or hospital knows you are the health care agent. Be prepared to bring or fax a copy of the health care power of attorney. (Email is not considered secure.) Keep a copy handy in your home or car, so you won't have to hunt for it in an emergency. Be sure you know where the original is located, so you can bring it, too, if requested.

- Don't be afraid to ask questions to make sure health care workers are honoring your loved one's wishes. Remind people firmly of those wishes as needed. Be as pleasant as possible, but don't back down.

- Make sure you understand your loved one's medical condition and the likely outcome. Sometimes doctors use unfamiliar terms. Ask them to explain in simpler terms until you fully understand the situation and options. Also make sure you and the doctors are speaking the same language. For example, your loved one may define "recovery" as living without the use of organ support like dialysis, but it may mean something else to the doctors.

- If you're wondering whether to start or stop a treatment, ask the doctor to discuss what you know about the patient's goals for care and priorities. Together, focus on how to translate these goals into a course of treatment. If the treatment fails, regroup and consider the next option.

- Treatment decisions often require you to weigh potential benefits versus burdens. Always think about what your loved one would consider a benefit or burden, not what you or anyone else might think.

- If diagnostic tests are recommended, ask what difference the results will make to treatment. If the impact will be little to nothing, the test may not be necessary, especially if it involves discomfort, risk, or excessive expense.

- If you feel your loved one's wishes are being ignored, talk to a social worker, patient representative, chief medical officer, or the institution's ethics committee or lawyer. As a health care agent, you are an advocate for someone who can't advocate for himself or herself. Don't be afraid to do whatever it takes to ensure that your loved one's wishes are recognized and respected.

- Recognize that some decisions are especially hard to make and might cause you to feel very sad, even if you feel you are carrying out wishes as planned.

- Part of your job as agent is to explain what is going on to other caring family members. Tactfully inform the family that you were designated by the patient as his or her spokesperson, so you are the ultimate decision maker, but you understand the concerns of others and will keep them all "in the loop." Often, it's useful for the health care team to hold a family meeting to share information and perspectives.

Make sure you understand your rights and responsibilities. For more information, consult the American Bar Association's publication *Making Health Care Decisions for Someone Else: A How-To Guide.* You can find a copy online at www.health.harvard.edu/ABA.

And if you do not yet have a complete copy of this Special Health Report, *Advance Care Planning: A guide to advance directives, living wills, and other strategies for communicating health care preferences,* you can order a copy by going to www.health.harvard.edu/LW.

Note: Harvard Health Publishing gives permission to buyers of this report to copy or share this page with potential health care agents.

Do whatever works best for you, but do it soon, and have these conversations more than once. Our priorities tend to change as our life circumstances change. Knowing your wishes will be carried out is comforting to you and a gift to loved ones, who won't have to go through the stress of wondering if they're doing the right thing. Research shows that both patients and families are more satisfied with care if they have engaged in the process and that families suffer less stress, depression, and anxiety if patients engaged in advance care planning prior to death.

Don't forget, though, that while talking about your wishes is important, you still should legally appoint an agent and, possibly, fill out a living will or POLST.

Privacy rules and health care agents

Since 2003, U.S. hospitals, doctors, and health plans have had to follow federal rules to keep patients' personal health information private. When you visit a new health care facility—for example, a doctor's office or hospital—you will receive information on these rules and be asked to sign a paper stating that you understand them. These privacy rules are part of a larger piece of legislation known as the Health Insurance Portability and Accountability Act, commonly referred to by the acronym HIPAA (pronounced HIP-uh).

HIPAA does not affect access to your doctor or your health care information by your health care agent when the proxy has been invoked. By signing the health care power of attorney form (or a similar state-specific form), you authorize your agent to gain access to your medical records and discuss your health care needs with your providers when he or she is acting as your proxy. In the legal language of HIPAA, your agent is your "personal representative."

In your advance directive, or in a separate document, you can also expressly identify family or friends with whom you want your health care providers to share medical information. This will not affect your agent's authority as the decision maker for you. And if you don't want your doctor to talk to certain people, you can make that clear in your directive. Be aware, however, that this means these individuals won't be able to get any information at all from the doctor.

Occasionally, people misinterpret the privacy rules. If a health care provider or anyone else tells you that he or she cannot share health information with an agent because of HIPAA, showing them the information from the HIPAA website may help. You can search different categories and questions online at the HIPAA Frequently Asked Questions page, which you can reach through www.health.harvard.edu/HIPAA. Alternatively, you can call the HIPAA toll-free hotline (see "Resources," page 46).

What if an adult patient who is sick and unable to communicate has no health care agent, and a family member wants to talk to the doctor or nurse? The HIPAA rules give health care providers discretion as to what is appropriate to disclose in this situation. Some providers are especially concerned about divulging information over the phone because they can't verify who is talking to them. But in most instances, the doctor should be able to discuss a patient's health status, treatment, or payment arrangements with the patient's family or close friends, unless the patient objects. This, too, is discussed on the HIPAA website. ⬮

STEP 3 · Creating your advance directives

Once you've chosen a health care agent and clarified your goals of care, you may be ready to translate your wishes into advance directives.

One option, short of creating a formal advance directive document, is to communicate your goals directly to your physician, who can summarize them in your medical record. As a practical matter, such an instruction will be limited to your immediate situation and will lack the portability of a formal directive. It will also lack some of the protections and visibility that a formal document provides. Or you can create a formal or informal document that states your wishes.

You can start the process of creating your advance directives by reading the information that follows on possible scenarios.

Working with scenarios

Knowing your health status today, it is possible for you to determine your goals for care (see "Step 1: Deciding on your wishes for care," page 8). But what if your health status suddenly changes—you get into a devastating accident or you suffer a massive stroke? Many states' living wills present several scenarios, then ask what types of care you would want in those situations if you were unable to make and voice your own decisions. Here are four scenarios often used:

1 You are likely to die within a short time, and organ-sustaining treatments would, at best, delay but not prevent death.

2 You have permanent and severe brain damage with no known hope of recovery, and organ-sustaining treatments would, at most, delay death.

3 You have brain damage and are in a coma from which you are not expected to awaken or recover, and organ-sustaining treatments would, at best, delay death.

4 You have reached an "end-stage condition" and your health is so poor you cannot mentally or physically care for yourself, and organ-sustaining treatments would, at most, delay death.

It is crucial to be aware that in all of these scenarios, the intent of organ-sustaining treatment is to prolong life, but it doesn't always work (and especially not in scenario 4).

The choices for care range from full-court press—that is, every treatment intended to keep you alive is offered, including CPR, ventilation, hemodialysis, artificial feeding, hydration, and others as needed—to choosing selectively among these options.

Many experts in the field are wary of using scenarios such as these in living wills. Why? They are too simplistic. Life rarely falls so neatly into place, and real medical situations may be much more complex. It's impossible to predict what will happen and what new options for care will be available. And it's hard to know how you will feel about certain treatments and quality-of-life issues when actually facing them.

"Stay flexible," urges Charles P. Sabatino, director of the American Bar Association's Commission on Law and Aging and legal editor of this report. "Never say never. I see people redraw the lines all the time as quality-of-life issues that seemed unacceptable in a state of health—being unable to feed or toilet themselves, for example—are reconsidered from a state of illness."

For this reason, it's good to frame your instructions as guidance, not mandates. You can do that simply by stating in the directive that the instructions given in the document are intended as guidance, and your agent has the authority to interpret or modify your instructions in order to carry out what he or she believes are your values and wishes. If you have a health care agent, make it clear to him or her that your wishes are to be treated as guidance, not binding instructions. Talk with your agent about conditions that you feel would make your quality of life unacceptable, such as an inability to recognize family members or sustaining severe, irreversible brain damage.

Who needs to have your advance directives?

Sometimes, people put living wills and health care power of attorney forms in a safe deposit box. That's safe if the house burns down, but won't be much help if you're unexpectedly hospitalized without them. Instead, take the following steps:

- Give your health care agent and any alternate agents a copy of your health care power of attorney (and your living will, if you have one). In an emergency, your agent may need to fax or email the documents to doctors or a hospital.
- Ask your doctor(s) to scan copies of directives into your electronic medical record or put paper copies of your directives into your file.
- If you are in the hospital, ask to have a copy of your directives put in your chart. (Your health care agent or a family member should do this if you are unable to do it.)
- File the original documents in a safe spot in your home (and tell your agent, family, and friends the location). Hospitals may ask to see an original, so it's important that people can find it when necessary. The National Hospice and Palliative Care Organization suggests writing the location of the original on the copies.
- Put a card in your wallet that displays your health care agent's name and contact information. Note where you keep the original and additional copies of the directive.
- Consider downloading a smartphone app such as Mind Your Loved Ones or MyDirectives to keep your documents accessible (see "Building more effective directives," below).
- If you are living at home and have a non-hospital

Building more effective directives

Even the best-prepared directive doesn't guarantee that everything will proceed as hoped when a crisis occurs.

An *Annals of Internal Medicine* editorial noted several hitches that commonly occur. These include inaccessible directives; agents who wilt under fire from other family members; and doctors who fail to comply with the directives, or who question whether the patient had the capacity to make sound decisions in the directive. Other research has shown that doctors frequently don't know there is an advance directive and that directives often aren't documented in patient charts.

Time will tell whether new approaches, such as POLST, and increasing use of electronic medical records can help solve these problems. In the meantime, having an advance directive still means you're much more likely to receive the treatment you want than if you don't make your wishes known.

In addition, these measures may help to ensure that your wishes are honored:

- Follow the instructions in this report for sharing copies of your directives (see "Who needs to have your advance directives?" above).
- Carry a wallet card with contact information for your agent and alternates, plus the location of the originals of your directives.
- Download a smartphone app, such as Mind Your Loved Ones or MyDirectives (see "Apps," page 47). Either app

will keep your advance directive and other documents accessible on your smartphone and transferable to your family members, friends, and health care personnel.

- Add your directives to your state's online registry, if available, or a national registry (see "National registries for advance directives," page 48).
- Talk to your doctor ahead of time and ask if he or she has any hesitations about your wishes or foresees possible conflicts. Make sure he or she enters your wishes in an electronic medical record, if available, or in your chart.
- Choose an agent based not on whom you love most, but on who you believe is most comfortable and reliable in taking on this taxing role. Consider who is most able to discuss your wishes with doctors and mediate conflicts.
- Ask family members if they are comfortable with your wishes. If you foresee major conflicts that you can't resolve, consider disqualifying certain people from making any care decisions by stating this in your health care power of attorney.
- Plan ahead with your agent. If you are ever hospitalized, he or she should bring or fax your directive to the hospital as soon as possible with a request that it go into your chart. (Email may or may not be accepted, as it is less secure.) Often, a fax can be sent to the attending physician or the nurses' station responsible for your care, although it's best to follow up to be sure it goes into your chart.

DNR or POLST form, remember that you or your health care agent may be required to display a signed form, or you may have to wear a special bracelet identifying a DNR decision.

- If a lawyer drew up your advance directives, he or she may keep a copy, too. Ask if this is the case and, if so, how long the copy will be kept in the files.

- Also consider using an advance directive registry to enable health care providers to gain access to your written wishes via the Internet. Your state may operate a registry, or you can use a national registry (see "National registries for advance directives," page 48). The registries may be free or may charge fees. Before choosing one, consider how

When someone you love won't create an advance directive

What if someone you love doesn't have an advance directive? That's common, although the underlying reasons may differ. Basic barriers include thinking that an advance directive isn't needed, not wanting to think about death or serious illness, not wanting to burden people, not knowing enough about advance directives and health care choices, needing help to fill out the forms, and lack of time with the doctor to discuss the matter. A person's ethnic or cultural background can also be a barrier: minorities tend to be more suspicious of health care providers and resistant to talking about or completing advance directives. According to AARP, African Americans in home health care and nursing homes are half as likely as whites to have advance directives.

To deal with this situation, try asking your loved one two simple questions, even if you think you know the answers.

- Do you have an advance directive?

- If not, why not?

See if the responses offer clues for ways to help. Some people believe that writing advance directives is bad luck or think it means they no longer want medical care.

As a first step, just focus on getting your loved one to name a health care agent. Point out that many health care decisions are made when people are temporarily unable to make their own decisions because of a treatable illness or injury. It is each individual's right to

forgo advance care planning, but people need to know that in the American health system that means they will receive maximal medical care if they fall seriously or even terminally ill.

The next step is to go a bit further. You might say you would feel better if you knew your loved one's wishes before any problems arise. Try: "I love you, and I wouldn't want to do anything you didn't agree with if you were ever unable to tell me what you wanted." Another way to approach it might be to ask, "What would be most important to you if you were seriously ill and not likely to recover?" Or, if the person "doesn't want to think about death," you can point out that you're really talking about quality of life near the end of life, not death, and promise to keep the conversation as brief as possible. If writing directives seems daunting, you could offer to help or to accompany the person on a visit to the doctor to discuss options. Or you might suggest making an audio or video recording of the person's wishes to give to the doctor.

If you still meet with refusal, don't push the issue too much on that occasion. Changing behavior takes time and, often, many conversations. A study of people 65 and older, published in the *Journal of the American Geriatrics Society*, noted that filling out advance directives is a multistep process to which familiar stages of behavioral change apply: precontemplation, contemplation, preparation, action, and maintenance. Study participants were

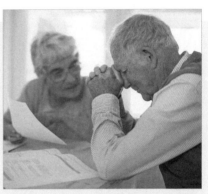

If your loved one "doesn't want to think about death," you can point out that you're really talking about quality of life near the end of life, not death.

likely to be at one stage for one step in the process—let's say, the completion of a health care agent form—and a different stage for another step, such as communicating with loved ones or clinicians about views on quality of life versus quantity of life. Another study in the same journal observed that older adults who had made decisions for someone at the end of life or witnessed this situation were more likely to participate in advance care planning for themselves.

Be willing to drop the subject of advance directives if your loved one gets angry or upset, but explain that you hope to discuss it another time. Then follow up. A news story or the experience of a relative or friend may provide the perfect opener. "Gee, here's what I'd want if that happened to me. What do you think you might want?" If you know your loved one's doctor or religious adviser, you can ask him or her for help. (For further advice, see "Pitfalls, fixes, and tips for tough conversations," page 27.)

© PeopleImages | Getty Images

access is granted to the documents and how much effort it will take to update them when necessary. Typically, a user name and password is required for security. This information can be kept on a wallet card, in the glove compartment of your car, and in your smartphone app, as well as given to appropriate people.

State-specific considerations

Advance directive forms vary from state to state. You can obtain a free copy of the current version of your state-specific advance directive from the National Hospice and Palliative Care Organization, through its CaringInfo program (for a shortcut, go to www. health.harvard.edu/nhpco). Many state bar associations and local hospitals also provide advance directive forms and information. If you do not have access to a computer or the Internet, try the public library. Most libraries provide free Internet access; you can ask a reference librarian for assistance.

Consult your state-specific form before filling out the health care power of attorney form in this report to find out any requirements, such as how many witnesses are needed and whether you need to get the document notarized. If you have questions about your state-specific information, call your local Area Agency on Aging or your Aging and Disability Resource Center. The Administration for Community Living (see "Resources," page 46) can help you find it. At this writing, all states and the District of Columbia permit an advance directive that combines a living will and health care agent appointment.

Here are some points to watch for as you look over your state rules:

- To create a legally binding directive, most states say you must be at least 18 years old (Alabama and Nebraska say 19 years old) and competent.
- It's wise to appoint alternate agents in case your primary choice is unavailable. State restrictions regarding choice of agent also apply to alternate agents.
- A health care power of attorney or living will does not necessarily prevent emergency medical personnel from performing CPR if your heart or breathing

▶ Do you need directives for two states?

Since different states recognize different documents, you may wonder if you need separate directives if you spend a lot of time in a second state. It's a reasonable question, but signing separate documents could actually complicate matters. When you sign a second advance directive, some states will deem that a revocation of the first directive. Plus, when documents are not worded the same, they may contradict each other.

If you spend a lot of time in another state, it's useful to obtain legal advice on how compatible the states' laws are. States normally will honor a directive that's validly signed in another state, although they may not have the same procedural rules for interpreting and implementing them. If you desire a different health care agent in the second state, that can be specified in a single health care power of attorney form.

stops. They are generally required by law to do so. If you do not wish to have CPR in an emergency, you must have a document signed by your doctor—either a non-hospital DNR or a POLST form—displayed in your home (usually on the refrigerator). Some out-of-hospital DNR protocols provide a bracelet to identify people with DNR orders.

- Some states require that you clearly note if you'd like your agent to have the power to reject or stop certain treatments such as artificial feeding and hydration. To avoid potential confusion, it is best to specify this authority on your advance directive no matter where you live.
- Witness requirements vary by state and sometimes include additional witnessing steps if you live in a health care facility.
- Notarization is not necessary in most states. In some states, you are permitted to use notarization as an alternative to having two witnesses.
- Procedures for changing or revoking an advance directive vary somewhat from state to state, but generally, you can revoke your document by destroying it, creating and signing a new advance directive, writing "Void" on the old document, or writing or stating your intent to revoke, and communicating your intent to revoke to your health care provider.

Religion-specific considerations

You may be concerned about whether your advance care plan is consistent with the tenets of your religious faith. All the major religions in the United States have endorsed the concept of advance directives, and many groups have developed sample directives to use in lieu of another directive, to supplement state-specific forms, or to guide surrogate decision makers.

The Christian Medical and Dental Societies provides information to help complete documents "in accordance with Biblical teaching and Christian tradition." Sample advance directives are available through Christian Life Resources and from many religiously affiliated health care systems within the United States.

The United States Conference of Catholic Bishops urges Catholics to consider designating a proxy decision maker in the event of incapacity and recommends choosing an agent who "understands and shares Catholic values." The organization accepts the use of DNR orders and advises Catholics to weigh the benefits and burdens of CPR to determine if it would constitute ordinary or extraordinary care.

The various branches of Judaism all advise designating a health care agent. Orthodox Jewish authorities advocate use of a Halachic Living Will (one that is consistent with traditional Jewish law) that includes the statement: "I hereby direct that all health care decisions made for me … be made pursuant to Jewish law and custom as determined in accordance with strict Orthodox interpretation and tradition." Such living wills include the name and contact information of an Orthodox rabbi who should be consulted by the health care agent to determine the requirements of Jewish law and custom.

The Islamic Medical Association of North America advocates that all Muslims draw up a living will and designate a health care surrogate. The sample living will recommended by the society's ethics committee includes language about allowing natural death in the event of terminal illness. It also specifically prohibits autopsy and requests burial in accordance with Islamic tradition.

You can generally obtain additional guidance about advance care planning and religion-specific forms from local churches, synagogues, and mosques.

Changing your advance care plan

Why revisit your advance care plan once you've completed it? Your goals of care may change over time. The American Bar Association Commission on Law and Aging suggests re-evaluating your advance care plans whenever any of the following "six D's" occurs:

- **Decade:** When you start each new decade of life.
- **Death:** When a loved one dies.
- **Divorce:** When you experience a divorce or other major family change. (In many states, a divorce automatically revokes the authority of a spouse who had been named as agent.)
- **Diagnosis:** When you are diagnosed with a serious medical problem.
- **Decline:** When you experience a significant decline from an existing health condition, especially when it diminishes your ability to live independently.
- **Domicile:** When you change your residence or when someone else moves in with you.

If you decide to change something in your living will or health care power of attorney, the best thing to do is create a new one. Once this new document is signed and dated in front of appropriate witnesses, and notarized if necessary, it supersedes your old directive.

To avoid confusion, make sure anyone who had a copy of your old directive gives it back to you so you can destroy it. Then distribute the new one (see "Who needs to have your advance directives?" on page 23). Remember to update directives stored in a registry, if you used one. And take the time to discuss these changes with your doctor and your health care agent to be sure everyone is on the same page. If you enter a nursing home or assisted living facility, make sure a copy of your advance directive gets filed in your medical records.

If you rely on any of the worksheets or decision-making tools we've described, you can revise them anytime you wish, but be sure to discuss the changes with your agent and any others who may be involved in making decisions on your behalf. ◆

Pitfalls, fixes, and tips for tough conversations

It's important to engage in advance care planning, but you may hit some roadblocks once you embark on the process. This chapter takes a look at a few common pitfalls and offers suggestions for how to avoid them. Hopefully, the scenes that follow will suggest words that may make tough conversations easier to start and continue.

Failing to choose a health care agent

The pitfall: Peter and Chris had been loving partners for four years. They talked about practically everything under the sun. One day, Peter had a car accident that sent him to the hospital with serious injuries. Because they weren't married, Chris could see Peter only during visiting hours. Much worse, Chris didn't have the authority to make important decisions for Peter's care, which fell instead to Peter's only living relative, a sister. She lived on the other side of the country and wasn't at all close to Peter or Chris. This could have been avoided if Peter had designated Chris as his health care agent.

The fix: Choose a health care agent and fill out the form. If you change your mind at a later date, you can name a different agent.

Choosing a health care agent, but never getting around to having "the conversation"

The pitfall: Dante asked Maria to be his health care agent, but somehow never got around to sharing his health goals and fears. When Dante developed complications after getting pneumonia and became unable to communicate, Maria was distraught. She had a hard time making decisions because she felt so unsure of what Dante would want.

Maria's experience is all too common. When an illness or accident strikes, people often feel stunned, surprised, and saddened. Meanwhile, real decisions must be made, sometimes urgently. When an agent has little or no guidance, it's terribly hard to deal with

an emotional response to the situation, yet clearly think through options.

The fix: Tell people what you want. If you haven't had this conversation because you aren't completely certain about what you want, that's okay. Try, at least, to talk about what your priorities or goals in living would be if you had a serious, potentially fatal condition.

If you're the health care agent, start asking right away, preferably before papers are signed. You can say, "I need to know what kind of care you'd want if you get really sick, or if there's some kind of catastrophe." Or, "We all really care about you. We love you and want to make sure you get the kind of care you want when you need it and can't tell us what you'd prefer. So that we won't have to guess—and maybe guess wrong, which would be awful—can we talk about what you'd want? What would be most important to you?" When the person finally agrees to talk, pull out the health decisions worksheet (see page 35) and go through it together.

Count on having more than one conversation. Try to be patient enough to consider "what if" questions even if the subject makes you anxious and upset. Check back every now and then—especially when an illness occurs or a decline in abilities is apparent—to decide if there has been any shift in goals. Sometimes people adapt to new limitations set by illness or accidents, which may prompt a change of heart about what makes life worth living.

Choosing the wrong person to be your health care agent

The pitfall: James and Kalinda had been married for 25 years. They agreed to engage in advance care planning after James had a serious heart attack that left him physically weakened for the rest of his life. Kalinda was fine with James being her health care agent and wanted to be his. But he feared that she wouldn't respect his wishes to not be resuscitated if he had another heart attack and preferred that his daughter serve as his health care agent. He didn't want to hurt Kalinda's feelings, however, so he chose her.

The fix: Talk to your family members and explain why you are choosing one person over another. Often spouses believe they must pick their partner or parents think they must choose one of their children, even if they have differing views on how much care they would wish to receive under certain dire circumstances. In this instance, it is important to stand your ground rather than give in—it could be the difference between dying peacefully and living for years with life-sustaining interventions against your wishes.

Making your wishes too broad or too specific

The pitfall: Rashid told Ellen he would never want to be on a ventilator—not in a million years, even if he was seriously ill. In fact, he was horrified by this prospect because his father had spent the last days of his life "hooked up to machines." Then he had a bad accident at work and ended up hospitalized, in a coma. His prognosis was reasonably good—the doctors felt it was likely he would come out of it. There was a catch, though. When Rashid was taken to the hospital, he was unconscious, and no one knew his wishes. His heart and breathing stopped, so CPR was performed. To stabilize him, the emergency team put him on a ventilator before Ellen arrived with a copy of Rashid's health care power of attorney. Ellen knew Rashid never wanted to be on a ventilator. However, she also realized that if Rashid had understood that a ventilator could be a bridge to a full recovery, he might have been more flexible in his wishes. Now she had to determine whether to have the doctors take him off the ventilator.

The fix: Avoid absolute instructions about specific treatments unless you are currently approaching a decision about the specific treatment. You might not fully understand the medical terms and implications of your choices. Have a conversation with your doctor as well as your health care agent about what you really want. A dialogue is more likely to turn up "what if" questions: What if a ventilator were needed as a bridge to recovery? Would it be all right to use it for a trial period if doctors thought it might help you regain consciousness?

If you're a health care agent, probe gently for more information. You needn't take "You know my wishes—don't keep me tied to machines and that's it!" as the final answer. Ask questions and listen carefully. "What is it you fear?" "What if there was a good chance that you could be returned to health?"

Having family members who disagree

The pitfall: Suzanne was dying. Now in the later stages of dementia, she could no longer eat or drink on her own. Suzanne had never appointed a health care agent, and her son, Henry, and her daughter, Cynthia, battled bitterly about appropriate treatment. Usually their opinions were 180° apart. Each insisted he or she knew their mother best and thus knew what she would have wanted.

"Should a feeding tube be placed?" the doctor asked.

"No," said Cynthia, believing that a feeding tube would only prolong death. "I know my mother wouldn't have wanted to live like this." Henry disagreed, saying their mother loved life and would want to live as long as she could. The disagreement had to be resolved through a consultation with the hospital ethics committee and intervention by a mediation lawyer. Ultimately, Suzanne did not have a feeding tube placed.

The fix: Name a health care agent now, while you are able to do so. Relatives may still argue, but your agent will have the legal authority to decide. When there's total gridlock and no one is willing to budge, people often go to court demanding to be named a legal guardian, a process that can take weeks and be very costly. A judge has to choose between the parties, or can decide to appoint a different guardian. Meanwhile, attention and energy better directed toward caring for the patient is pulled into the conflict. The patient gets lost in the shuffle, and everyone on the hospital team must tread water while the family hashes it out in court.

If you've chosen a health care agent, you may be able to head off serious disagreements by sharing your wishes with everyone in the family. If you know ahead of time that someone is likely to vehemently object, you can choose to disqualify that person from weighing in on medical decisions by writing that instruction in your directives. ◆

The forms

In this section, you'll find five key forms, along with tips for filling them out:
- **Form 1:** Health care power of attorney
- **Form 2:** Health decisions worksheet
- **Form 3:** Generic living will
- **Form 4:** Sample POLST form.

Tips for filling out your directives

Do the following before you sit down to fill out your directives:

- Use the health decisions worksheet (Form 2, page 35) to sort out your thoughts on end-of-life issues and think about your goals for care and priorities. The worksheet is not intended to be a formal advance directive but rather a tool to provide meaningful guidance for your decision makers.
- Decide which forms you wish to fill out and copy or download state-specific versions of these forms.
- Read all instructions carefully.
- You don't need a lawyer to help you fill out the forms, but you do need witnesses to sign the forms after you complete them. Check on the correct number of witnesses required and be prepared to have the form notarized, if that is required in your state. Some states permit notarization as a substitute for two witnesses.
- If you are appointing a health care agent, you can use the health care power of attorney form in this report (Form 1, page 30), which is usually accepted, or obtain a state-specific health care power of attorney form through your doctor. Alternatively, you can download one from CaringInfo, a website of the National Hospice and Palliative Care Organization (go to www.health.harvard.edu/nhpco).
- If you choose to write a living will, you can use our generic living will (Form 3, page 39), or get a state-specific form through your doctor or download one

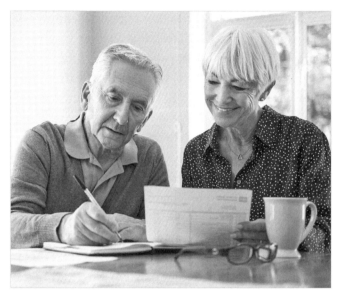

The first step in creating advance directives is to sort out your thoughts on end-of-life issues. Then decide which forms you want to fill out, and print out versions that are accepted in your state.

from CaringInfo (go to www.health.harvard.edu/nhpco). Different state forms ask different questions, but most cover similar topics and leave room for you to write in requests not covered.

- If you have a serious, life-limiting disease, are significantly weakened and experiencing difficulty with daily tasks because of frailty, and are at risk of dying within the next year or two, you may choose to fill out a state-specific POLST/POST/MOLST/MOST form, available at www.polst.org/educational-resources/resource-library or by searching on the Internet for your state's form. (The specifics and name of the form may vary, and the POLST is still in development in many states, so availability could change from moment to moment.)
- Distribute copies of your advance directives to the appropriate people. See "Who needs to have your advance directives?" on page 23 for further guidance on where to store your directives and who to give them to.

Download a PDF version of this form at **www.health.harvard.edu/ADforms**.

This form allows you, the principal, to name a person to make health care decisions for you if you are unable to do so. You should also name alternate agents in case your first agent is unavailable or unwilling to serve.

This is a general form provided for your convenience. While it meets the legal requirements of most states, it may or may not fit the requirements of your particular state. Many states have special forms or special procedures for creating advance directives, which you can find at www.health.harvard.edu/nhpco. Even if your state's law does not recognize this document, it may still provide clear evidence of your wishes if you cannot speak for yourself.

Generally, it's not advisable to add overly specific instructions to your agent in this particular document because this can limit his or her ability to respond as you would want in the face of complex medical circumstances. If you include instructions, clearly state that they are intended only as guidance. Alternatively, try to give your agent as much guidance as you feel comfortable giving through conversations, the health decisions worksheet (Form 2, page 35), or both.

Directions

Fill in names, addresses, and contact information. After deciding which decisions you want your agent to be able to make, cross out and initial any that you do not wish to include. Be sure to comply with state requirements for agents (and witnesses, if needed). Depending on whether your state requires witnesses or notarization, or both, you must meet these rules so that the document will be valid. In a few states, your agent may be asked to sign an acceptance or acknowledgement form before acting as agent.

See "Who needs to have your advance directives?" on page 23 for guidance on where to store your directives and whom to give copies to.

Requirements for agents

To comply with most of the legal variations across all the states, your agent should be at least 18 years old (19 in Alabama and Nebraska) and should not be

- your health care provider, including the owner or operator of a health or residential or community care facility serving you
- an employee (or spouse of an employee) of your health care provider
- serving as health care agent for 10 or more people.

For more information, go to www.health.harvard.edu/state-limits.

Requirements for witnesses

Some states allow notarization as an alternative to two witnesses. Each state has rules regarding witness disqualification (that is, who cannot serve as a witness to sign these documents). Check your own state's requirements, but to cover virtually all variations in state law, choose witnesses who are at least 18 years old (19 years old in Alabama and Nebraska) and who are not

- the individual appointed as agent or alternate agent
- related to you by blood, marriage, or adoption
- your health care provider, including the owner or operator of a health, long-term care, or other residential or community care facility serving you
- an employee of your health care provider
- financially responsible for your health care
- an employee of your life or health insurance provider
- a creditor of yours or entitled to any part of your estate under a will or codicil, by operation of law
- entitled to benefit financially in any other way during your life or as a result of your death.

I, _____ ıt

Print your name here as it appears on your driver's license or birth certificate

ıt.

_____

Agent's name

_____

Agent's address

_____

Phone numbers, fax number, email address

If this person is unwilling, unable, or unavailable to act, or if I revoke his or her appointment, I designate the following person to act for me in making my health and medical decisions:

_____

Name of first alternate agent

_____

Address

_____

Phone numbers, fax number, email address

If neither of the above people is available, or if I revoke both of their appointments, my next choice is:

_____

Name of second alternate agent

_____

Address

_____

Phone numbers, fax number, email address

This power of attorney shall become effective when I am no longer able to make health care decisions. This requirement will be met whenever it has been determined by one or more doctors that I cannot provide informed consent. If my state requires a different procedure, then the state's procedure should be followed. My agent shall have full authority to make health and medical decisions for me, according to what he or she thinks I would have wanted, based on any written or verbal communication we have had on the subject, other written communication I may have left, and any verbal communication I have made to others if my agent has reason to believe they are accurate statements of my preferences. I intend my agent's authority to interpret my wishes to be as broad as possible.

If a decision needs to be made on a matter about which I have left no reliable guidance, my agent shall decide what he or she thinks is in my best interests, consistent with my values, goals, and priorities as understood by my agent. My agent's authority should include, but not be limited to, the ability to do the following. I have crossed out and initialed any statements I do not want to include:

- Consent to, refuse, or withdraw consent to any and all types of treatments, services, tests, surgeries, and care. These include but are not limited to artificial respiration (including ventilator care), artificial nutrition and hydration, dialysis, organ transplantation, and medications. This authority includes decisions that could or would allow my death.

- Request or consent to the issuance of a do-not-resuscitate order (DNR) by my attending physician, which would forgo cardiopulmonary resuscitation (CPR) when CPR will provide no benefit to me, as determined by my physician.

- Authorize admission or discharge from nursing homes, hospitals, assisted living facilities, or other similar facilities, even against medical advice if he or she believes it is what I would have wanted.

- Have the same access to medical records and information as I am entitled to, including the ability to disclose information to others.

- Hire and fire medical, health care, or support personnel as needed.

- Take any legal action needed to ensure my wishes are followed.

- Move me to another state, if need be, to carry out my wishes or to get me the care I need.

- Consent to any medications or treatments intended to provide comfort care and relieve pain, even if such actions may cause physical dependence, lead to physical damage, or hasten the moment of (but not intentionally cause) my death.

- Sign any waiver or release forms necessary.

- Authorize my participation in medical research.

- To the extent permitted by law, make decisions about organ donation, autopsy, and disposition of remains, even after my death.

Here I list any additional instructions to my agent:

_____

_____

_____

_____

_____

_____

_____

_____   _____
Signature   Date

Witnesses

I have witnessed that the principal has signed this document in my presence while he or she was of sound mind, and not under undue influence, constraint, or duress.

I also declare that I am over 18 years of age (19 in Alabama and Nebraska) and am NOT

- the individual appointed herein as agent or alternate agent
- related to the principal by blood, marriage, or adoption
- the principal's health care provider, including owner or operator of a health, long-term care, or other residential or community care facility serving the principal
- an employee of the principal's health care provider
- financially responsible for the principal's health care
- an employee of the principal's life or health insurance provider
- a creditor of the principal or entitled to any part of the principal's estate under a will or codicil, by operation of law
- entitled to benefit financially in any other way while the principal lives or as a result of the principal's death.

Witness signature #1

Printed name of witness

Address

Phone numbers, fax number, email address

Witness signature #2

Printed name of witness

Address

Phone numbers, fax number, email address

Notarization

Many states permit notarization as an alternative to two witnesses. Notarization or notarization plus two witnesses is required only in certain states. Check with the state in which you live to find out if this applies to you. Or simply go the extra step and use two witnesses and a notary to cover all possibilities.

State of _____ County of _____

On this _____ day of _____ , 20 _____ , the said _____ ,

known to me (or satisfactorily proven) to be the person named in the foregoing instrument, personally appeared before me, a Notary Public, within and for the State and County aforesaid, and acknowledged that he or she freely and voluntarily executed the same for the purposes stated therein.

My commission expires: _____

Notary Public _____

Download a PDF version of this form at **www.health.harvard.edu/ADforms**.

This worksheet is presented for your convenience to help you consider and explain your goals for care. Understanding your values and priorities gives everyone valuable information about the kind of care you would and would not want in different situations. Your answers can help you start a conversation with your doctor, health care agent, and loved ones.

While your state's law probably will not legally recognize this document as an advance directive, it will still provide important evidence of your wishes if you cannot speak for yourself. It will help guide your agent and anyone else with whom you share this worksheet. If you like, you can transfer the information to a state-specific living will form, too (see "State-specific considerations," page 25).

Directions

The questions in this directive will help you describe your goals for care, end-of-life thoughts and preferences, and decisions about comfort care and organ donation. Alternatively, you can fill out your preferences for care by using the scenarios in our generic living will (Form 3, page 39). Read both forms first to decide which approach will work best for you.

Feel free to jot down thoughts in complete sentences or in fragments, whichever is more comfortable for you. You may find you don't have answers for some of the questions. If you need more space, use another sheet of paper. (For definitions of the various medical procedures and terms, see "Understanding key medical procedures and programs," page 12, and "Medical terms, to know," page 16.) Revisit these questions if your medical status or other important matters change. Once you've completed the form, see "Who needs to have your advance directives?" on page 23 for guidance on where to store your directives and who to give copies to.

_____   _____
Name of person completing this worksheet   Date

Thoughts and preferences

In general, how do I feel about the final stage of life? What do I think my fears will be? What do I think will bring me the most joy?

_____

_____

_____

If I had only a short time to live, what would my most important priorities be?

_____

_____

_____

Is there anyone I would not want to be involved in discussions or decisions about my care?

_____

_____

Where and how would I like to spend the last days of my life? At home? In a hospital?

_____

_____

_____

Would I like music played or particular items kept near me?

_____

_____

_____

Would I like lots of visitors? Just a few?

_____

When I am close to death, would I like a religious leader called to my bedside? ❑ Yes ❑ No
Who else would I like to have notified?

_____

_____

Medical care

In general, what are my goals in the event of a serious, progressive illness? For example, do I want treatment aimed at keeping me alive as long as possible under any circumstances, regardless of the side effects of the treatment? Do I want exclusive focus on my comfort? Do I only want treatments that are unlikely to compromise my daily function (activities such as hearing, walking, talking, and reading)? How do I prioritize these goals?

_____

_____

Most people imagine a serious illness as far in the future. Would my answer to the previous question change if I were hit by a car tomorrow? (Be cautious. Research tells us that some people become more accepting of illness and disability once they experience it.)

_____

If I were unconscious and unable to hear, feel, think, talk, or eat, and my doctors said I had little hope of recovery:

- Would I want artificial nutrition (tube feeding)? ❑ Yes ❑ No
- Would I would want artificial hydration? ❑ Yes ❑ No
- Would I want to be kept alive by a mechanical ventilator, assuming I was unable to breathe on my own?
  ❑ Yes ❑ No

If I were unconscious, and unable to hear, feel, think, talk, or eat, and doctors said I had a chance of recovery:

- Would I want to try artificial nutrition (tube feeding) for a trial period if my doctor thought it might help me regain consciousness?   ❏ Yes   ❏ No
- Would I want it stopped if it failed to help?   ❏ Yes   ❏ No
- Would I want to try artificial hydration for a trial period if my doctor thought it might help me regain consciousness?   ❏ Yes   ❏ No
- Would I want it stopped if it failed to help?   ❏ Yes   ❏ No
- If I were unable to breathe on my own, would I want to be kept alive by a mechanical ventilator for a trial period if my doctor thought it might help me regain consciousness?   ❏ Yes   ❏ No
- Would I want it stopped if it failed to help?   ❏ Yes   ❏ No

Notes: _____

_____

If I had severe brain damage (say, I could neither speak nor understand what was going on around me) and was not expected to recover:

- Would I want to be kept alive by machines, such as a mechanical ventilator, and receive artificial nutrition (tube feeding), artificial hydration, and any other measures intended to keep me alive?   ❏ Yes   ❏ No

Notes: _____

_____

What, if anything, bothers me about being kept alive by machines?

_____

_____

How much weight do I give the opinions of doctors? Of my family members?

_____

_____

Before making medical decisions on my behalf, I would like my health care agent, if I have appointed one, to consult with the people named below. However, my agent will have the right to overrule the opinions of other people, even those I have asked him or her to consult.

_____

_____

Do I have any religious or spiritual beliefs that should guide doctors and others responsible for making decisions about my care?

_____

_____

What are my biggest concerns or fears regarding care near the end of life?

_____

_____

Comfort care

Under what circumstances would I want other treatments stopped and comfort care initiated?

_____

_____

_____

_____

Which symptoms, if any, particularly concern me (for example, pain, anxiety, nausea, or shortness of breath)?

_____

_____

_____

_____

Organ and tissue donation

Would I like to be an organ and tissue donor (check one)?

❏ No. I do not wish to donate organs or tissue.

❏ Yes. I would like to donate any organ and tissue.

❏ Yes. I would like to donate only the following organs or tissue:

_____

_____

I want my donation, if any, to be for the following purposes (check one):

❏ Transplant or research

❏ Transplant only

❏ Research only

Download a PDF version of this form at **www.health.harvard.edu/ADforms.**

We have provided this generic living will form, which contains four scenarios, for your convenience. If you also fill out the health decisions worksheet (Form 2, page 35), be very careful that your instructions in the two documents match, so that you do not create confusion for your caregivers and health care agent.

While this generic living will form meets the legal requirements of most states, it may or may not fit the requirements of your particular state. **It is very important that you use a form that meets the requirements of your own state.** This one is adapted from the Oregon form, but many states have special forms or special procedures for creating health care advance directives. You can find your own state's form at www.health.harvard.edu/nhpco. Even if your state's law does not recognize the document in this report, it will still provide important evidence of your wishes if you cannot speak for yourself. In other words, it would serve as an advisory document, even if not a legal document.

Directions

You, the principal, should fill in your name, address, and contact information. Depending on whether your state requires witnesses or notarization, or both, you must meet these rules so that the document will be valid. After reading through each of the four scenarios, check boxes next to the options. We recommend discussing the scenarios with your doctor, who can help you make choices that reflect your values and beliefs. Add notes for further clarification, if you like. All scenarios assume you are unable to voice your wishes.

Once you've completed the form, see "Who needs to have your advance directives?" on page 23 for guidance on where to store your directives and who to give copies to.

Requirements for witnesses or notarization

Most states require the signatures of two witnesses on a living will; some allow notarization of the document instead. Three states—Missouri, South Carolina, and West Virginia—require both notarization and two witnesses.

Each state has rules regarding witness disqualification (that is, who cannot serve as a witness to sign these documents). Check your own state's requirements, but to cover virtually all variations in state law, choose witnesses who are at least 18 years old (19 years old in Alabama and Nebraska) and who are *not*

- the individual you've appointed as your health care agent or an alternate agent
- related to you by blood, marriage, or adoption
- your health care provider, including the owner or operator of a health, long-term care, or other residential or community care facility serving you
- an employee of your health care provider

- financially responsible for your health care
- an employee of your life or health insurance provider
- a creditor of yours or entitled to any part of your estate under a will or codicil, by operation of law
- entitled to benefit financially in any other way while you are living or as a result of your death.

Your name

_____

Address

_____

Phone numbers, fax number, email address

_____

Birth date

This living will shall become effective upon disability or incapacity of the principal. This requirement will be met whenever it has been determined by one or more doctors that I cannot provide informed consent, or when I meet all the requirements for effectiveness mandated by state law.

If my state requires a different procedure, then my state's procedure should be followed.

Health care instructions

Note: In filling out these instructions, keep the following in mind:

- The term "as my physician recommends" means that you want the physician treating you to try life support if your physician believes it could be helpful and then discontinue it if it is not helping your health condition or symptoms.

- "Life support" refers to any medical means for keeping you alive, including procedures, devices, and medications. If you refuse life support, you will still get routine measures to keep you clean and comfortable.

- "Tube feeding" refers to food and water supplied artificially by medical device. If you refuse tube feeding, you should understand that death will probably result.

- You will get care for your comfort and cleanliness, no matter what choices you make.

- You may either give specific instructions by filling out items 1 to 4 below, or you may use the general instruction provided by item 5.

Here are my desires about my health care if my doctor and another knowledgeable doctor confirm that I am in a medical condition described below:

1. Close to death. If I am close to death and life support would only postpone the moment of my death:

A. Initial one:

_____ I want to receive tube feeding.

_____ I want tube feeding only as my physician recommends.

_____ I DO NOT WANT tube feeding.

B. Initial one:

_____ I want any other life support that may apply.

_____ I want life support only as my physician recommends.

_____ I want NO life support.

2. Permanently unconscious. If I am unconscious and it is very unlikely that I will ever become conscious again:

A. Initial one:

_____ I want to receive tube feeding.

_____ I want tube feeding only as my physician recommends.

_____ I DO NOT WANT tube feeding.

B. Initial one:

_____ I want any other life support that may apply.

_____ I want life support only as my physician recommends.

_____ I want NO life support.

3. Advanced progressive illness. If I have a progressive illness that will be fatal and is in an advanced stage, and I am consistently and permanently unable to communicate by any means, swallow food and water safely, care for myself, and recognize my family and other people, and it is very unlikely that my condition will substantially improve:

A. Initial one:

_____ I want to receive tube feeding.

_____ I want tube feeding only as my physician recommends.

_____ I DO NOT WANT tube feeding.

B. Initial one:

_____ I want any other life support that may apply.

_____ I want life support only as my physician recommends.

_____ I want NO life support.

4. Extraordinary suffering. If life support would not help my medical condition and would make me suffer permanent and severe pain:

A. Initial one:

_____ I want to receive tube feeding.

_____ I want tube feeding only as my physician recommends.

_____ I DO NOT WANT tube feeding.

B. Initial one:

_____ I want any other life support that may apply.

_____ I want life support only as my physician recommends.

_____ I want NO life support.

5. General instruction.

Initial if this applies:

_____ I do not want my life to be prolonged by life support. I also do not want tube feeding as life support. I want my doctors to allow me to die naturally if my doctor and another knowledgeable doctor confirm that I am in any of the medical conditions listed in Items 1 to 4 above.

6. Additional conditions or instructions. Insert description of what you want done.

_____

_____

_____

_____   _____

Signature   Date

Declaration of witnesses

We declare that the person signing this advance directive

- is personally known to us or has provided proof of identity

- signed or acknowledged that person's signature on the advance directive in our presence

- appears to be of sound mind and not under duress, fraud, or undue influence

- has not appointed either of us as a health care representative or alternate representative

- is not a patient for whom either of us is the attending physician.

_____   _____
Witness signature #1   Date

_____
Printed name of witness

_____
Phone number, email address

_____   _____
Witness signature #2   Date

_____
Printed name of witness

_____
Phone number, email address

Note: For restrictions on who can serve as a witness, see page 1 of this form.
Adapted with permission from the Oregon Advance Directive Form.

Download a PDF version of this form at **www.health.harvard.edu/ADforms**.

Each state that provides for physician orders for life-sustaining treatment (POLST) has its own form and its own name for the form (POLST, MOLST, POST, or MOST). In this report, we have provided the new National POLST form issued by the National POLST Paradigm Task Force. At this writing, no state has yet adopted the national form. The task force published it to serve as a model for states and coax them toward more uniformity in their POLST documents.

If your physician completes a POLST form for you, it will have to be the version of the form that's recognized in your state. More than half the states have POLST programs in place, and most of the remaining states are in various stages of developing a POLST program. You can find a link to your state-specific POLST form online in the resource library of the National POLST Paradigm Task Force at www.polst.org/educational-resources/resource-library; select "Forms" under "Resource type." State programs that meet voluntary national standards are referred to as "endorsed" programs and are identified at www.polst.org.

Because POLST is a medical order, it must be filled out and signed by a physician or other authorized professional, working in close collaboration with you, so that you have a thorough understanding of your current medical circumstances and your treatment options in the event of an emergency, and your doctor has a thorough understanding of your priorities and goals of care.

Remember: POLST is appropriate only for individuals with serious, progressive illnesses or frailty who are at risk of dying within the next year.

HIPAA PERMITS DISCLOSURE OF POLST ORDERS TO HEALTH CARE PROVIDERS AS NECESSARY FOR TREATMENT
SEND FORM WITH PATIENT WHENEVER TRANSFERRED OR DISCHARGED

Medical Record # (Optional)

National POLST Form: A Portable Medical Order

Health care providers should complete this form only after a conversation with their patient or the patient's representative. The POLST decision-making process is for patients who are at risk for a life-threatening clinical event because they have a serious life-limiting medical condition, which may include advanced frailty (www.polst.org/guidance-appropriate-patients-pdf).

Patient Information.	**Having a POLST form is always voluntary.**
This is a medical order, not an advance directive. For information about POLST and to understand this document, visit: www.polst.org/form	Patient First Name: _____ Middle Name/Initial: _____ Preferred name: _____ Last Name: _____ Suffix (Jr, Sr, etc): _____ DOB (mm/dd/yyyy): ___/___/_____ State where form was completed: _____ Gender: ☐ M ☐ F ☐ X Social Security Number's last 4 digits (optional): xxx-xx-__ __ __ __

A. Cardiopulmonary Resuscitation Orders. Follow these orders if patient has no pulse and is not breathing.

Pick 1

☐ YES CPR: Attempt Resuscitation, including mechanical ventilation, defibrillation and cardioversion. (Requires choosing Full Treatments in Section B)

☐ NO CPR: Do Not Attempt Resuscitation. (May choose any option in Section B)

B. Initial Treatment Orders. Follow these orders if patient has a pulse and/or is breathing.

Reassess and discuss interventions with patient or patient representative regularly to ensure treatments are meeting patient's care goals. Consider a time-trial of interventions based on goals and specific outcomes.

Pick 1

☐ **Full Treatments (required if choose CPR in Section A).** Goal: Attempt to sustain life by all medically effective means. Provide appropriate medical and surgical treatments as indicated to attempt to prolong life, including intensive care.

☐ **Selective Treatments.** Goal: Attempt to restore function while avoiding intensive care and resuscitation efforts (ventilator, defibrillation and cardioversion). May use non-invasive positive airway pressure, antibiotics and IV fluids as indicated. Avoid intensive care. Transfer to hospital if treatment needs cannot be met in current location.

☐ **Comfort-focused Treatments.** Goal: Maximize comfort through symptom management; allow natural death. Use oxygen, suction and manual treatment of airway obstruction as needed for comfort. Avoid treatments listed in full or select treatments unless consistent with comfort goal. Transfer to hospital **only** if comfort cannot be achieved in current setting.

C. Additional Orders or Instructions. These orders are in addition to those above (e.g., blood products, dialysis).
[EMS protocols may limit emergency responder ability to act on orders in this section.]

D. Medically Assisted Nutrition (Offer food by mouth if desired by patient, safe and tolerated)

Pick 1

☐ Provide feeding through new or existing surgically-placed tubes ☐ No artificial means of nutrition desired

☐ Trial period for artificial nutrition but no surgically-placed tubes ☐ Discussed but no decision made (standard of care provided)

E. SIGNATURE: Patient or Patient Representative (eSigned documents are valid)

I understand this form is voluntary. I have discussed my treatment options and goals of care with my provider. If signing as the patient's representative, the treatments are consistent with the patient's known wishes and in their best interest.

✖ (required)

If other than patient, print full name:		Authority:	The most recently completed valid POLST form supersedes all previously completed POLST forms.

F. SIGNATURE: Health Care Provider (eSigned documents are valid) Verbal orders are acceptable with follow up signature.

I have discussed this order with the patient or his/her representative. The orders reflect the patient's known wishes, to the best of my knowledge. [Note: Only licensed health care providers authorized by law to sign POLST form in state where completed may sign this order]

✖ (required)

	Date (mm/dd/yyyy): Required ___/___/_____	Phone # : ( )
Printed Full Name:		License/Cert. #:
Supervising physician signature: ☐ N/A		License #:

A copied, faxed or electronic version of this form is a legal and valid medical order. This form does not expire. 2019

Courtesy of National POLST

National POLST Form – Page 2   *****ATTACH TO PAGE 1*******

Patient Full Name:

Contact Information (Optional but helpful)

Patient's Emergency Contact. (Note: Listing a person here does **not** grant them authority to be a legal representative. Only an advance directive or state law can grant that authority.)

| Full Name: | ☐ Legal Representative
☐ Other emergency contact | Phone #:
Day: (   )
Night: (   ) |

Primary Care Provider Name: Phone:
                                                                                                                        (   )

☐ Patient is enrolled in hospice   Name of Agency:
                                                                    Agency Phone: (   )

Form Completion Information (Optional but helpful)

Reviewed patient's advance directive to confirm no conflict with POLST orders:
(A POLST form does not replace an advance directive or living will)

☐ Yes; date of the document reviewed:_____
☐ Conflict exists, notified patient (if patient lacks capacity, noted in chart)
☐ Advance directive not available
☐ No advance directive exists

Check everyone who participated in discussion: ☐ Patient with decision-making capacity ☐ Court Appointed Guardian ☐ Parent of Minor
☐ Legal Surrogate / Health Care Agent   ☐ Other:_____

Professional Assisting Health Care Provider w/ Form Completion (if applicable):
Full Name: Date (mm/dd/yyyy): /   /   Phone #: (   )

This individual is the patient's: ☐ Social Worker ☐ Nurse ☐ Clergy ☐ Other:

Form Information & Instructions

- Completing a POLST form:
  - Provider should document basis for this form in the patient's medical record notes.
  - Patient representative is determined by applicable state law and, in accordance with state law, may be able execute or void this POLST form only if the patient lacks decision-making capacity.
  - Only licensed health care providers authorized to sign POLST forms in their state or D.C. can sign this form. See www.polst.org/state-signature-requirements-pdf for who is authorized in each state and D.C.
  - Original (if available) is given to patient; provider keeps a copy in medical record.
  - Last 4 digits of SSN are optional but can help identify / match a patient to their form.
  - If a translated POLST form is used during conversation, attach the translation to the signed English form.
- Using a POLST form:
  - Any incomplete section of POLST creates no presumption about patient's preferences for treatment. Provide standard of care.
  - No defibrillator (including automated external defibrillators) or chest compressions should be used if "No CPR" is chosen.
  - For all options, use medication by any appropriate route, positioning, wound care and other measures to relieve pain and suffering.
- Reviewing a POLST form: This form does not expire but should be reviewed whenever the patient:
    (1) is transferred from one care setting or level to another;
    (2) has a substantial change in health status;
    (3) changes primary provider; or
    (4) changes his/her treatment preferences or goals of care.
- Modifying a POLST form: This form cannot be modified. If changes are needed, void form and complete a new POLST form.
- Voiding a POLST form:
  - If a patient or patient representative (for patients lacking capacity) wants to void the form: destroy paper form and contact patient's health care provider to void orders in patient's medical record (and POLST registry, if applicable). State law may limit patient representative authority to void.
  - For health care providers: destroy patient copy (if possible), note in patient record form is voided and notify registries (if applicable).
- Additional Forms. Can be obtained by going to www.polst.org/form
- As permitted by law, this form may be added to a secure electronic registry so health care providers can find it.

| State Specific Info | For Barcodes / ID Sticker |

For more information, visit www.polst.org or email info@polst.org   Copied, faxed or electronic versions of this form are legal and valid.   2019

Resources

Organizations

AARP
601 E St. NW
Washington, DC 20049
888-687-2277 (toll-free)
www.aarp.org

AARP is a nonprofit, nonpartisan organization that addresses the needs and interests of people ages 50 and older. Its website has abundant information on end-of-life issues.

Administration for Community Living
330 C St. SW
Washington, DC 20201
202-401-4634
800-677-1116 (toll-free Eldercare Locator)
www.acl.gov

This government umbrella agency oversees Administration on Aging programs across the country. Through the Eldercare Locator, it offers a wide range of information and local services for older adults and their families or caregivers, including contact information for the nearest Area Agency on Aging, state-specific advance directives, transportation, in-home help, adult day care, and support groups.

American Bar Association Commission on Law and Aging
1050 Connecticut Ave. NW, Suite 400
Washington, DC 20036
202-662-8690
www.americanbar.org/groups/law_aging

The ABA Commission on Law and Aging, headed by Charles P. Sabatino, legal editor of this report, offers information from experts on health law, advance care planning, and other issues, as well as links to agencies and experts who can help with legal issues in your state. The website includes a section on legal and medical matters relating to older adults, as well as current and past issues of *Bifocal*, the commission's bimonthly journal, which contains a wealth of legal resources and information you can read for free.

CaringInfo (formerly Caring Connections)
National Hospice Foundation
1731 King St., Suite 100
Alexandria, VA 22314
800-658-8898 (toll-free)
www.caringinfo.org

Part of the National Hospice and Palliative Care Organization, this program provides free bilingual resources and information to help people make decisions about end-of-life care and services, including state-specific forms for living wills and health care power of attorney.

Donate Life America
701 E. Byrd St., 16th Floor
Richmond, VA 23219
804-377-3580
www.donatelife.net

This not-for-profit alliance of national organizations and local coalitions across the United States educates the public about organ and tissue donation. The organization provides forms and information on how to become an organ donor as well as an online registry.

National Hospice and Palliative Care Organization
1731 King St., Suite 100
Alexandria, VA 22314
800-658-8898
www.nhpco.org

This nonprofit organization represents hospice and palliative care programs and experts across America. Hospice care aims to enhance quality of life in many realms for patients (and their caregivers) during the last six months of life. Palliative care seeks to address physical, emotional, social, and spiritual pain for all patients and families. The NHPCO website and HelpLine offer publications on these topics and can provide information on locating programs.

National POLST Paradigm (Physician Orders for Life-Sustaining Treatment)
c/o Emmer Consulting, Inc.
208 I St. NE
Washington, DC 20002
202-780-8352
www.polst.org

This national organization created and disseminates information on POLST, a set of prepared medical orders for people with life-limiting conditions that is designed to work in a full range of care settings, including emergency care, hospitals, nursing facilities, and home care. The orders, which complement but do not replace advance directives, are created by an individual in consultation with health care providers, and signed by the person's physician, giving the orders added weight in emergency situations.

U.S. Dept. of Health and Human Services Office for Civil Rights
200 Independence Ave. SW
Washington, DC 20201
800-368-1019 (toll-free)
www.hhs.gov/hipaa

This federal office, part of the U.S. Department of Health and Human Services, administers the Health Insurance Portability and Accountability Act (HIPAA), which protects the privacy of personal health information. The HIPAA website provides details on the rules governing access to your information by your health care agent and others involved in your care.

Publications

Being Mortal: Medicine and What Matters in the End
Atul Gawande, M.D., M.P.H.
(Metropolitan Books, 2014)

In this groundbreaking treatise, Harvard University surgeon Atul Gawande, a frequent contributor to *The New Yorker*, proposes reversing the medical trend toward providing maximal care to extend life in the elderly and seriously ill. Rather, he argues, we should emphasize death with dignity, while preserving quality of life and honoring a dying patient's wishes and goals.

The Conversation: A Revolutionary Plan for End-of-Life Care
Angelo E. Volandes, M.D.
(Bloomsbury, 2016)

This Harvard physician and researcher offers the stories of seven patients and their different journeys through end-of-life care. To improve this inevitable stage of life, he advocates a plan that revolves around conversations between physicians and patients. The goal is to empower patients to live out their last days in the way they want to, and not the way the medical system dictates.

The Denial of Aging: Perpetual Youth, Eternal Life, and Other Dangerous Fantasies
Muriel Gillick, M.D.
(Harvard University Press, 2007)

In one of the earliest books to critique the American medical system's preoccupation with holding off the aging process by providing maximal testing, drugs, and procedures to prolong life at any cost, Dr. Muriel Gillick, medical editor of this report, argues for treatment that is geared to achieving a person's goals of care. She emphasizes the role of "intermediate care" near the end of life for many patients—health care that focuses on quality rather than quantity of life. The book is anchored by stories from Dr. Gillick's clinical experience as a geriatrician and palliative care physician, her advice to accept the inevitability of aging, and her guidance for caregivers.

Dying in America: Improving Quality and Honoring Individual Preferences Near the End of Life
Institute of Medicine of the National Academies Committee on Approaching Death: Addressing Key End-of-Life Issues
(National Academies Press, 2015; available for free download at www.nap.edu/catalog/18748)

This comprehensive review of research evidence, including results of an Institute of Medicine study about current attitudes and practices around end-of-life care in the United States, is primarily for health care providers, policy makers, and researchers. However, it contains a wealth of information on a "good end" to life, including the value of advance care planning, for interested consumers.

Handbook for Mortals: Guidance for People Facing Serious Illness
Joanne Lynn, M.D., Joan Harrold, M.D., and Janice Lynch Schuster
(Oxford University Press, 2011)

A comprehensive and readable guide to dealing with serious, eventually fatal illness and the final years of life.

Jane Brody's Guide to the Great Beyond: A Practical Primer to Help You and Your Loved Ones Prepare Medically, Legally, and Emotionally for the End of Life
Jane Brody
(Random House, 2009)

Jane Brody, a long-time health columnist for *The New York Times*,

presents a pragmatic, wide-ranging book delving into end-of-life care. Topics discussed include advance directives, caregiving, hospice and palliative care, spirituality, and what to say or leave unsaid.

A Life Worth Living: A Doctor's Reflections on Illness in a High-Tech Era
Robert Martensen, M.D.
(Farrar, Straus, and Giroux, 2008)

A thoughtful, provocative book from a physician, historian, and bioethicist. Dr. Martensen reflects on end-of-life issues, delving into what gives life meaning and considering ways in which never-ending options for extended care affect us as individuals and as a society.

Making Medical Decisions for Someone Else: A How-To Guide
The American Bar Association Commission on Law and Aging
(ABA, 2009; you can find it at www.health.harvard.edu/ABA)

This free handbook from the ABA was created to assist people who have been tasked with making health care decisions for another person. It covers the different kinds of health care proxies—health care agent, legal surrogate, and guardian—that can be appointed, the medical decisions and common scenarios you might face, ways of working within the health care system, and advice for resolving disputes and getting help.

Apps

Mind Your Loved Ones (MYLO)
American Bar Association

This mobile app gives individuals and their family members the ability to store their own and each other's health care directives, critical medical information, and other related data on a phone. This information then can be sent directly to health care providers by fax, email, or text. Users can share information and profiles. The app is available on a subscription basis from Google Play and Apple App Store.

MyDirectives MOBILE
ADVault, Inc.

This app enables you to create a document using your iPhone, iPad, or iPodTouch that combines a living will and a health care power of attorney. The information is kept in an online registry and can be accessed by your health care providers right on the lock screen of your phone, or send it by email, text, or QR code. You also can express your preferences about resuscitation, organ donation, and autopsy. The app makes it possible to record a video of your wishes and include emergency contact information. It is available from the Apple App Store.

Online tools

Advance Planning for Dementia
https://dementia-directive.org

This free online tool can help you think through what kind of care you would want to receive if you had mild, moderate, or severe dementia.

The Conversation Project
www.theconversationproject.org

A multimedia website focused on helping people talk to loved ones and doctors about desires for end-of-life care.

Five Wishes
www.fivewishes.org

This very simply written advance directive helps record personal, spiritual, and emotional wishes for the end of life as well as medical ones. Five Wishes has been translated into many languages.

MyDirectives
https://mydirectives.com

This online tool allows you to create a document that combines a living will and a health care power of attorney, which can be accessed by your health care providers.

National Healthcare Decisions Day
www.nhdd.org

Held annually in April, National Healthcare Decisions Day provides a great opportunity to discuss advance care planning with loved ones.

Prepare for Your Care
https://prepareforyourcare.org

Available in English or Spanish, the website of this nonprofit organization takes you through a free, step-by-step process to think through your needs and preferences about end-of-life care.

Webcast

Thorough and thoughtful coverage on end-of-life issues has been produced in a variety of media. Here is one excellent webcast available for download at the time this report was being written:

End of Life Care in America: A Doctor's Diagnosis
www.health.harvard.edu/martensen

Robert Martensen, author of *A Life Worth Living: A Doctor's Reflections on Illness in a High-Tech Era*, speaks to Terry Gross on Fresh Air, a National Public Radio program, about many issues surrounding medical care and final illnesses.

National registries for advance directives

Several national registries will store advance directives electronically so that health care providers have access to your wishes. Below are two options. As of this writing, 11 states also have their own registries. They are Arizona, California, Idaho, Michigan, Montana, Nevada, North Carolina, Oklahoma, Vermont, Virginia, and West Virginia.

America Living Will Registry
www.alwr.com

U.S. Advance Care Plan Registry
www.usacpr.net

Glossary

advance care planning: The process involved in learning about and deciding upon the kinds of care you wish to receive if you are too ill or incapacitated to make medical decisions yourself, then communicating these wishes to your doctor and loved ones.

advance directive: A legal document that allows you to describe the kind of medical care you hope to receive and who you want to speak for you if an accident or illness renders you unable to communicate. Two examples are the health care power of attorney and the living will.

artificial nutrition: A procedure that supplies nutrients and fluids via a tube that goes into the stomach (inserted through the nose or the abdominal wall) or intravenously, though a vein.

artificial respiration: A procedure that may be performed during CPR in which a plastic mask placed over the mouth and nose is attached to a tube and bag. The bag is squeezed and released, moving air in and out of the lungs of a person who has stopped breathing.

autopsy: Examination of a body externally and internally after death; typically performed to determine the cause of death.

brain death: Typically, an irreversible state of unconsciousness in which the heart still beats but the person demonstrates a lack of reflexes and deliberate movements, cannot breathe without help from a machine, and has no electrical activity in the brain. Exact legal definitions of brain death vary by state.

cardiopulmonary resuscitation (CPR): A procedure aimed at reviving a person whose heart or breathing has stopped.

coma: A deep, sleeplike state of unconsciousness from which a person cannot be aroused.

comfort care: A broad term that may encompass medication, oxygen, and a variety of equipment or efforts aimed at relieving troubling symptoms, such as pain, labored breathing, anxiety, and other forms of physical or emotional discomfort. Sometimes called intensive comfort care or palliative care.

defibrillation: An electric shock delivered to the body by a medical device called a defibrillator in order to reset an abnormal heart rhythm to a normal, steady rhythm. Frequently used during CPR.

do-not-resuscitate order (DNR): A medical order written by a physician reflecting a patient's wishes that hospital staff not perform CPR if the person's heart or breathing stops. Also called a do-not-attempt-resuscitation order (DNAR) or allow-natural-death order (AND).

electronic medical record: Computerized medical records used by some hospitals and health care facilities, which are replacing paper charts in certain states and health care settings.

guardian: A person or agency appointed by the court system to make health care and legal decisions for another person. The guardian is accountable to the court that appoints him or her. Also called a conservator.

health care agent: The person chosen by you to make medical decisions on your behalf when you are unable to make these decisions yourself because of illness or incapacitation. Also called a health care proxy, surrogate, or health care representative, among other titles.

health care power of attorney: A legal document that enables you to name a person to act as your health care agent to make medical decisions on your behalf when you are unable to do so because of illness or incapacitation. Also called a health care proxy form, medical power of attorney, durable power of attorney for health care, or appointment of a health care representative form.

hemodialysis: The use of a machine or system that filters blood to help maintain the right balance of fluids and essential minerals and clear away wastes.

hospice: A program designed to deliver comprehensive comfort care when curative treatments can no longer help or further treatment seems futile.

intravenous hydration: Fluids given through a tube connected to a needle that is inserted into a vein.

living will: A legal document that enables people to express their wishes about the kinds of medical care they would like to receive, or would like to avoid, if they are unable to communicate their wishes directly because of illness or incapacitation.

mechanical ventilation: A procedure to assist breathing using a tube inserted through the nose, mouth, or throat into the trachea (windpipe) and attached to a machine called a ventilator, or respirator, which pushes air into and out of the lungs.

minimally conscious state: A state of impaired consciousness marked by occasional moments of awareness, such as smiling or crying in response to emotional stimuli, vocalizing, making purposeful sounds, or reaching for objects.

non-hospital DNR: A medical order available in some states to complement a standard DNR. This form, which directs emergency personnel not to perform CPR if the person's heart or breathing stops, may be used in the home or at an assisted living facility or nursing home. Also called out-of-hospital DNR order.

organ donation or tissue donation: Surgical removal of healthy organs or tissues after death, to be transplanted into another person.

palliative care: Supportive care that addresses symptom relief, psychological issues such as depression, family conflict, caregiver guilt, and advance care planning for people with serious advanced illnesses and their family members. It can be given concurrently with life-prolonging care or as a component of hospice care.

physician orders for life-sustaining treatment (POLST): A portable medical order signed by a physician after a voluntary process of shared, informed decision making with an individual and reflecting the person's values and goals for care. The order addresses what to do in the event of an emergency when decisions need to be made quickly about CPR, whether to transport to the hospital, comfort care versus full treatment, and the use of artificial nutrition and hydration. POLST is intended for people who have serious life-limiting medical conditions, which may include advanced frailty. Also known as physician orders for scope of treatment (POST), medical orders for life-sustaining treatment (MOLST) or medical orders for scope of treatment (MOST). These orders do not substitute for naming a health care agent.

principal: The legal term for the person who names another to act as his or her agent.

terminally ill: Having an advanced illness or condition that cannot be cured and can ultimately lead to death. Frequently, use of the term indicates that a limited span of months, weeks, or days are expected before death.

vegetative state: A state of impaired consciousness in which a person appears to be awake with eyes open. Breathing and heartbeat continue because the brainstem is working, yet other brain functions, such as thought, speech, and purposeful movement, have ceased.

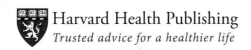 **Harvard Health Publishing**
Trusted advice for a healthier life

 Receive *HEALTHbeat*, Harvard Health Publishing's free email newsletter

Go to: **www.health.harvard.edu** to subscribe to *HEALTHbeat*. This free weekly email newsletter brings you health tips, advice, and information on a wide range of topics.

You can also join in discussion with experts from Harvard Health Publishing and folks like you on a variety of health topics, medical news, and views by reading the Harvard Health Blog (**www.health.harvard.edu/blog**).

Order this report and other publications from Harvard Medical School

online	|	**www.health.harvard.edu**
phone	|	877-649-9457 (toll-free)
mail	|	Belvoir Media Group Attn: Harvard Health Publishing P.O. Box 5656 Norwalk, CT 06856-5656

Licensing, bulk rates, or corporate sales

email	|	**HHP_licensing@hms.harvard.edu**
online	|	**www.health.harvard.edu/licensing**

Other publications from Harvard Medical School

Special Health Reports *Harvard Medical School publishes in-depth reports on a wide range of health topics, including:*

Addiction	Eye Disease	Osteoporosis
Advance Care Planning	Foot Care	Pain Relief
Aging in Place	Grief & Loss	Positive Psychology
Allergies	Hands	Prostate Disease
Alzheimer's Disease	Headaches	Rheumatoid Arthritis
Anxiety & Stress Disorders	Hearing Loss	Sensitive Gut
Back Pain	Heart Disease	Sexuality
Balance	Heart Disease & Diet	Skin Care
Cardio Exercise	Heart Failure	Sleep
Caregiving	High Blood Pressure	Starting to Exercise
Change Made Easy	Incontinence	Strength Training
Cholesterol	Joint Pain Relief	Stress Management
Cognitive Fitness	Knees & Hips	Stretching
COPD	Life After Cancer	Stroke
Core Workout	Living Longer	Tai Chi
Depression	Memory	Thyroid Disease
Diabetes	Men's Health	Vitamins & Minerals
Diabetes & Diet	Mobility & Independence	Walking for Health
Energy/Fatigue	Neck Pain	Weight Loss
Erectile Dysfunction	Nutrition	Women's Health
Exercise	Osteoarthritis	Yoga

Periodicals *Monthly newsletters and annual publications, including:*

Harvard Health Letter	*Harvard Heart Letter*	*Prostate Disease Annual*
Harvard Women's Health Watch	*Harvard Men's Health Watch*	

ISBN 9781614012382

52900

ISBN 978-1-61401-238-2
SX66000

LW1119